Comments on C̶h̶r̶o̶n̶i̶c̶ ̶O̶b̶s̶t̶r̶u̶c̶t̶i̶v̶e̶ ̶P̶u̶l̶m̶o̶n̶a̶r̶y̶ Disease – the
'at your fingertip' guide from readers

Comments on **Chronic Obstructive Pulmonary Disease – the
'at your fingertips' guide** from *reviewers*

'The book is excellent and I wish you every success with it.'
*Dr A C Miller, Consultant Physician
Mayday University Hospital, Croydon, Surrey*

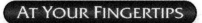

CHRONIC OBSTRUCTIVE PULMONARY DISEASE

Dr Jon Miles MD, MEd, FRCP
Consultant Physician, North Manchester General Hospital
Facilitator, Education for Health, Warwick
Associate Postgraduate Dean, North Western Deanery

June Roberts SRN, DipHE (PN), FETC, DipAsthma, DipCOPD,
DipAllergy
Nurse Practitioner, Langworthy Medical Practice, Salford
Honorary Research Fellow, University of Aberdeen
Facilitator, Education for Health, Warwick

CLASS PUBLISHING • LONDON

Printing history
First published 2005
Reprinted with revisions 2006

10 9 8 7 6 5 4 3 2

The authors and the publisher welcome feedback from the users of this book. Please contact the publisher.

Class Publishing (London) Ltd
Barb House, Barb Mews,
London W6 7PA
Telephone: 020 7371 2119
Fax: 020 7371 2878 [International +4420]
Email: post@class.co.uk

The information presented in this book is accurate and current to the best of the authors' knowledge. The authors and publisher, however, make no guarantee as to, and assume no responsibility for, the correctness, sufficiency or completeness of such information or recommendation. The reader is advised to consult a doctor regarding all aspects of individual health care.

A CIP catalogue record for this book is available from the British Library.

ISBN-10: 1 85959 045 4
ISBN-13: 978-1-85959-045-4

Edited by Gillian Clarke
Indexed by Valerie Elliston
Cartoons by Jane Taylor
Drawings by Andy Roberts
Line diagrams by David Woodroffe
Typeset by Sally Brock
Printed and bound in Finland by WS Bookwell, Juva

Contents

Foreword

by Professor Peter M A Calverley, MB, FRCP, FRCPE
Professor of Medicine (Pulmonary and Rehabilitation),
University of Liverpool

Chronic obstructive pulmonary disease (COPD) is gradually shedding its Cinderella image and is at last being recognised as a widespread cause of disability and premature death in the UK. For many years it was possible to dismiss the complaints of people with COPD as being 'just bronchitis' and to assume that it was just a matter of time before the reduced number of smokers in the population led to this disease disappearing.

Many people have successfully stopped smoking and avoided a premature death from smoking-related illnesses but, as they age, the damage they did to their lungs earlier catches up with them and they develop symptoms of cough sputum and particularly persistent breathlessness that limit their lives and prevent them from achieving all that they could wish. Hence the need for better care for people with COPD and a wider recognition of how it creeps up on them and limits their lives.

Whilst doctors in general and even the UK Government have become better at addressing these problems, there is still a shortage of accessible information for people who are affected by this terrible condition. Thankfully, this book helps bridge the gap between the patients and their carers by providing authoritative and up-to-date information about almost all aspects of COPD diagnosis and care. Patients often feel that they do not have time to ask all the questions that they need answering when they see the specialist nurse, GP or hospital specialist. This book will provide them with background information to help them understand what is wrong with them and how it might be treated.

We know that this is a condition that is best prevented, and if this is not possible then COPD usually requires more than just one form of treatment. The authors have taken a comprehensive view of both drug and physical therapy and emphasise the positive steps that patients themselves can take to help them to cope with this illness. We are making progress in our fight against the enormous problems that COPD presents. Hopefully, as more progress occurs, future editions of this book will be needed. Certainly it gives the general reader an easily accessible way of getting to grips with the common but often misunderstood condition.

Acknowledgements

We are grateful to the many people who have helped with the book, in particular:

Professor Peter Calverley, for finding the time in his very busy schedule to write the Foreword

Rachel Booker and Monica Fletcher, of the National Respiratory Training Centre, for all their help and advice

Jane Scullion, of Glenfield Hospital, Leicester, for help and suggestions

Jean Whitworth, for reading the manuscript and commenting on it from the patient's point of view

Dr A C Miller for reviewing the book for us

The British Lung Foundation's Breathe Easy groups, for telling us what people want to know

Chest, Heart and Stroke of Scotland, for telling us what people want to know

The National Respiratory Training Centre, for permission to use their diagrams and instructions on the use of inhalers

Stefan Cembrowicz and Theresa Allain, for the basis of a number of answers in the 'Getting help' chapter, from *Osteoporosis – the 'at your fingertips' guide*

Class Publishing for recognising the undoubted need for a patient's book on COPD

Andy Roberts, with Mark Smith, for the new illustrations

and, of course, our patients who provided many of the questions for us to answer.

And last but not least, Hat and Charlie and the rest of our families for putting up with us.

Introduction

For years, chronic obstructive pulmonary disease (COPD) was regarded with some disdain by health-care professionals. It was considered to be a disease that was largely self-inflicted and that sufferers almost 'got what they deserved'! Fortunately, attitudes have changed a great deal and the whole approach to smoking-related lung disease is more positive and becoming increasingly proactive. In addition, people increasingly want to become involved in decisions about their own health care, and to do that they require the knowledge to enable them to ask the correct questions. *Chronic Obstructive Pulmonary Disease* is our attempt to equip people with COPD with the tools to do this. It is set out in a question-and-answer format and draws on the considerable experience we have gained in looking after people with COPD.

We dedicate this work to the many people with COPD with whom we have been involved and hope that it will provide a source of information and inspiration for many others.

Jon Miles and June Roberts

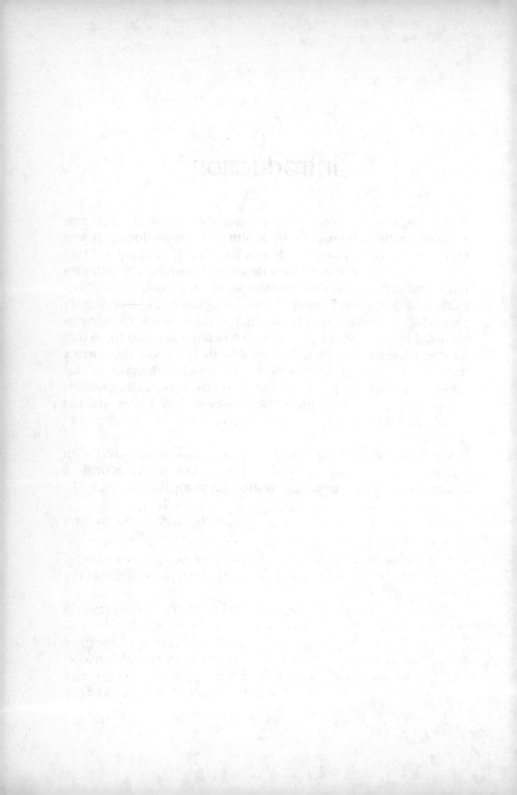

1
What is COPD?

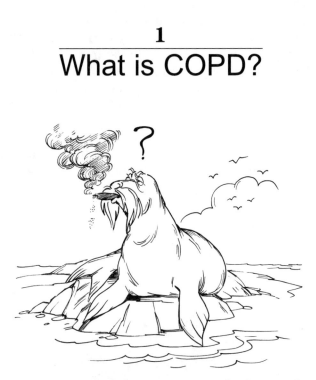

There are so many different terms, aren't there – bronchitis, asthma, emphysema, chronic obstructive pulmonary disease (COPD), chronic obstructive airways disease (COAD) and chronic obstructive lung disease (COLD). They all seem to be interchangeable and you will be forgiven for being very confused about them. So we will begin by explaining the reasons for all the different names.

It is only relatively recently that we have begun to understand the reasons why people develop lung diseases, and by this time some of the names mentioned above had already come into regular use. Most of the terms used are associated with narrowing of the air passages. Emphysema is the only exception because it is a condition that affects the tiny air sacs (the alveoli) in the lungs. So let's start with a bit of information about the role of the lungs in breathing.

The purpose of breathing is, first, to get oxygen from the air into the bloodstream so that it can help in the chemical reactions that help our other organs and muscles work properly. Breathing also allows us to remove carbon dioxide from the bloodstream. Carbon dioxide is a 'waste product' resulting from the functioning of our organs and muscles. As you can see from Figure 1.1, the airways provide the transport for these two gases to and from the lungs, and the alveoli are where oxygen is taken in and carbon dioxide is taken out of the bloodstream. If this system is damaged in any way, the process of breathing will be impaired and cause symptoms such as breathlessness and cough.

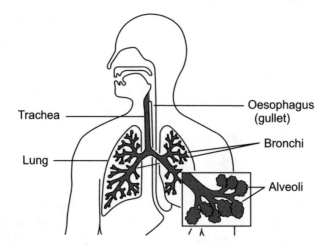

Figure 1.1 The breathing process

Definitions

Asthma and the others

The first major distinction, when it comes to the 'names', is to try to separate asthma from the rest. This is dealt with in more detail in Chapter 3 (***How is COPD diagnosed?***), but asthma is a condition that affects *only* the airways, is usually reversible and is caused mainly by allergies. It is common in children (affecting up to one in four children in some parts of the world), and can change in its nature throughout someone's life – being bad some days and almost not noticeable on others. If properly treated, asthma does not usually cause persistent narrowing of the airways. Occasionally, however, the disease can be so severe that people are disabled by it on a daily basis, resulting in major restrictions on their lifestyle.

Bronchitis and the others

Bronchitis literally means airway ('bronchi') inflammation ('itis'). It can affect people for just a short period of time, when it's called *acute bronchitis*, or it can go on for years, when it is known as *chronic bronchitis*. Probably nearly all of us have had acute bronchitis at some point in our lives: it usually follows a virus infection or cold and causes coughing, occasionally with some phlegm too. It usually lasts for only a week or two. By contrast, chronic bronchitis is a more specific condition and is defined by the amount of phlegm the person coughs up and the period over which this continues. To be diagnosed as having chronic bronchitis, you have to cough up phlegm every morning for at least three consecutive months within a period of at least two years. We shall see in Chapter 2 (***Work and the environment***) that a number of environmental influences may affect people with chronic bronchitis but the overwhelming cause of chronic bronchitis is cigarette smoking. The precise way that cigarettes do their damage is not known but we do know that it is unusual for people to develop chronic bronchitis without having been exposed to cigarette smoke.

Emphysema and the others

Most people have known someone who has been told they have emphysema. It is nearly always a person who has smoked heavily for a good many years, and such people are often very breathless.

Unlike conditions such as asthma and bronchitis, emphysema affects the alveoli – where the exchange of oxygen for carbon dioxide (*gas exchange*) takes place. As you can see in Figure 1.2, the alveoli are the air sacs where oxygen and carbon dioxide travel to and from the bloodstream; they are made of very elastic tissue so that they can expand and contract to let air in and out. This is usually an efficient process because we have millions of alveoli, all lying right beside very tiny blood vessels. In emphysema, large numbers of these alveoli have been destroyed and there is much less area for the gases to change places. So, although people can breathe the oxygen in, it cannot get into the bloodstream.

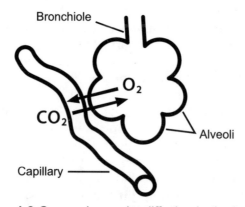

Figure 1.2 Gas exchange by diffusion in the lungs

My GP and practice nurse use lots of abbreviations when they're talking to me but 'COPD' is the main one. So what is COPD?

COPD stands for **C**hronic **O**bstructive **P**ulmonary **D**isease. It is also referred to as chronic obstructive airways disease (COAD) and chronic obstructive lung disease (COLD), but for the purposes of this book we are going to stick with COPD. If your doctor or nurse uses COAD or COLD, do not worry because the terms are pretty much identical. It's just that COPD has become the most widely used phrase, both in the UK and abroad. It is a name that tries to cover the effects of cigarette smoking on the lungs but does not include lung cancer. It has become an important term, because we now realise that many people have varying combinations of bronchitis and emphysema, and that some people with asthma also smoke and develop COPD.

Many different countries now have their own definitions of COPD but they all state that the characteristics of COPD are:

- narrowing of the airways,
- it does not change very much from day to day,
- it is likely to get progressively worse as the years go by.

This definition is important because it means that you can only be diagnosed as having COPD if you do a special breathing test (see Chapter 3, *How is COPD diagnosed?*).

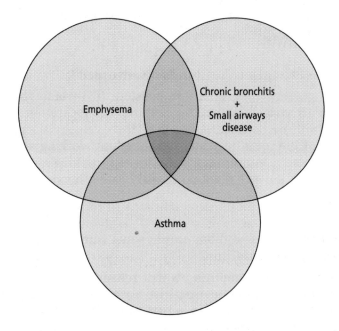

Figure 1.3 Diagrammatic representation of the overlap between chronic bronchitis, emphysema and asthma

I still don't really understand what my problem is. Do I have emphysema or not?

To be honest, emphysema can only be diagnosed by looking at specimens of your lung tissue under the microscope. This is not usually done because it doesn't really affect the care that you receive. Breathing tests in combination with a chest x-ray can give your doctor the information that will indicate whether you have emphysema; if you are experiencing symptoms such as breathlessness, the doctor may well start you on inhalers to try to improve your symptoms (see Chapter 6, *Inhalers and nebulisers*).

Although it is helpful to get as clear a picture of your illness as possible, the really important issue is whether you have damaged your lungs and air passages as a consequence of smoking cigarettes and what the best treatments are to help you. The treatments that are available at present that are likely to help you do not depend on your doctor knowing the exact nature of the damage to your lungs and air passages. However, this may change in the future.

Can the changes to my lungs be reversed?

At the present time it is not possible to reverse the damage caused to your lungs by such things as cigarettes, and your doctor will be concentrating on trying to maximise the performance of the parts of your lungs that are working well. This is why it is vitally important for you to stop smoking as soon as possible if you haven't done so already (see Chapter 4, *Stopping smoking*).

My father suffered from emphysema but he was a smoker. Does it run in families?

There is a form of emphysema that runs in families and is due to the lungs having low amounts of a protein called alpha-1 antitrypsin (AAT). This protein is part of the body's natural defence against particles we breathe in. It is very rare, though, and if you do not smoke it is unlikely that you will get emphysema even if other members of your family have had it.

The information you've given me is helpful but I'm still not sure whether to ask my GP for a test for this alpha-1 antitrypsin protein!

Remember that this deficiency is very rare. If, however, emphysema is diagnosed in a family member before the age of 40 years and you are suffering from breathlessness yourself, it may be worth discussing this with your GP. Again, the most important thing you can do is to stop smoking if you are currently doing so.

COPD and its symptoms

What are the symptoms of COPD? How do I know whether I've got it?

COPD affects both the airways and the lungs, so the most common symptoms are:

- cough – often associated with the production of phlegm,
- breathlessness – often limiting your ability to do things,
- wheeze – the noisy breath sounds that occur when the airways are narrowed.

Not everybody has all these symptoms. For example, some people first notice just a morning cough – the cough is often worse first thing in the morning. If you cough up phlegm, it is usually a white or light yellow colour. If the phlegm turns a darker yellow or increases in amount, this could mean that you have an infection and you should consult your GP. Breathlessness can be caused either by airway narrowing, limiting the flow of air into the lungs, or by damage to the air sacs, which leads to a problem with getting oxygen into the bloodstream. People often notice it first when they are trying to exercise – going upstairs, doing the shopping, walking up hill or that sort of thing – but there are people with severe COPD who are breathless even at rest (for more about severe COPD, see

Chapter 3, *How is COPD diagnosed?*). There are some other symptoms and signs associated with COPD, such as a feeling of chest tightness and ankle swelling, but, if you begin to experience any aches or pains or notice any features that are unusual for you, it is important that you mention these to the doctor or nurse.

So does everyone with a cough have COPD, then?

No, this is not the case. COPD is almost always associated with a long history of smoking cigarettes, so if you have never been a smoker it is very unlikely that your cough is due to COPD. Also, people who smoke can cough for reasons other than COPD. For example, coughing up blood or phlegm with specks of blood can sometimes be a result of having pneumonia, or a more permanent scarring condition of the lungs called *bronchiectasis*, or even something more serious such as a cancer of the lung. If you ever cough up blood or blood-specked phlegm, you should immediately make an appointment to see your doctor as you will probably require an x-ray of your chest to find out why this is happening.

I seem to be breathless compared with my mates. How do I know whether this is because of COPD?

Well, the truth is that you do not! This is why it is important to see your doctor so that the cause of your breathlessness can be determined. If you have been a smoker for a number of years, and have noticed a cough in the mornings where you bring up phlegm and that you have also been wheezy, it is possible that you have COPD. But remember that it will require a breathing test to confirm this diagnosis.

Also remember that people who smoke are also at an increased risk of heart disease. If your heart is not working well or is not getting enough oxygen due to narrowing of the arteries that supply it with blood, this can also make you breathless. The message is: if you are more breathless than your mates, you should be trying to find out why!

Is COPD catching? Can I give it to my children?

To say that something is 'catching' normally means it is 'infectious'. COPD cannot be passed on in this way. It is usually a response of your lungs to the effects of cigarette smoke. Of course, the other members of your household can potentially be affected by the cigarettes you smoke (passive smoking). We're afraid that there will be a regular important message occurring throughout this book: if you are a smoker *PLEASE STOP!*

The doctor tells me that I have COPD. Can COPD be cured?

Not as such, because some of the damage caused cannot be reversed. But it is possible to receive treatments that will make you feel better, and stopping smoking removes the primary cause in over 90 per cent of people with COPD. In addition, stopping smoking will stop you getting worse (see Figure 1.4)! An example of a treatment that is likely to help is being sure you get your yearly vaccine against influenza, as this will reduce the potential for you to be unwell over the winter period. There is more about the different treatments for COPD in Chapter 5.

Will having COPD affect my sex life?

In general terms there should not be a problem with your sex life. Obviously if you are prone to getting out of breath when you exercise, you may become breathless during intercourse! The only other problem that can affect men is that some of the treatments for COPD can affect your libido (see Chapter 9, *Living with COPD*). If you find that you are having problems in this area, please do not keep it to yourself but discuss it with your doctor or nurse: there are now a variety of treatments available to help.

Causes of COPD

I know loads of people who smoke and don't seem to have any trouble at all. So why have I got COPD?

We know – this can be very frustrating! The statistics show that about one in five people who smoke are likely to develop COPD. So it won't be uncommon for you to know people who have smoked a lot but haven't developed the condition. (They are quite likely to develop some of the other problems associated with cigarettes, though, such as heart attack, stroke and cancer!). The precise reason for this phenomenon is not clear. Some people think that there is an association between a person's genetic make-up and the effects of cigarette smoke. Some recent research has suggested that the lungs of far more than one in five people are affected by cigarette smoke but that the changes are too subtle to give people the symptoms of COPD. If you are one of the people affected in this way by cigarette smoking, the sooner you stop the better.

Figure 1.4 shows that your lungs function less well after about the age of 30 whether you smoke or not, but that the smokers suffer much worse than the non-smokers (compare the two black lines). Stopping smoking can partially halt this decline (look at the dashed lines coming off the solid line) – it is never too late to give up smoking!

There must be some other causes of COPD – surely!

OK, we know we've bombarded you with facts about smoking – and we're afraid that there's still a lot more to come. But, yes, there are some other things that might make it more likely for people to develop COPD. We'll go through them in turn.

INCREASING AGE

COPD comes on slowly, so it's unlikely to affect people until they are in their 40s or 50s. If you are under 40 and have been diagnosed with COPD, particularly if it runs in your family, you may need to be tested for a deficiency of the protein alpha-1 anti-trypsin in your lungs (discussed earlier).

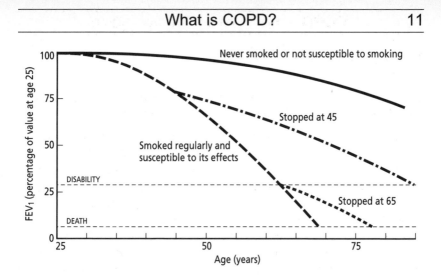

Figure 1.4 Decline in lung function as part of the normal ageing process and as accelerated by cigarette smoking. (Reproduced, with permission, from C. Fletcher and R. Peto, 1977, 'The natural history of chronic airflow obstruction. *British Medical Journal*, 1, 1645–8)

GENDER

COPD is more likely to affect men than women, although recent statistics show that women are catching up. The explanation is probably that the effects of smoking are being seen earlier in men and will show themselves in women soon. In fact, some people think that women are more susceptible to the effects of cigarette smoke. It is also likely that more women are smoking nowadays.

SOCIAL CLASS

COPD is more common in people in lower social class groups. It is thought that this is simply due to the different smoking rates in the various groups of people, and recently much attention has been paid to the effects of passive smoking (breathing in somebody else's cigarette smoke) on lung development. Another factor that may be important, and is also found in lower social class groups, is having been a small baby. Low birth weight can be associated with poor lung function in adult life. The airways develop during the first 16 weeks of pregnancy and the air sacs (alveoli) develop during the last few weeks of pregnancy and the first few years of life. Poor nutrition or severe infections occurring during this period (both these things are more common in lower social class groups) may affect the development of the lungs.

OCCUPATION

Some jobs have been associated with COPD. Coal mining has been the most publicised, but some welders and cotton workers also believe that their work has contributed to the development of COPD. We talk more about this in Chapter 2 (**Work and the environment**).

DIET

If you go into any health food shop these days you can find lots of information about *antioxidants*. These are substances that are thought to help the body to 'mop up' harmful things we breathe in (or eat) and prevent damage from occurring to our healthy cells. An example of antioxidants is vitamin C. An increasing number of people believe that antioxidants are particularly helpful at combating the effects of cigarette smoke. *BUT* nobody believes that taking antioxidants can mean it is OK to carry on smoking!

AIR POLLUTION

Since the industrial revolution, living in the city has always been associated with a greater tendency to getting chest complaints. Whilst this is true, whether pollution causes COPD or just makes existing COPD worse remains controversial. Again, there is more about this in Chapter 2.

But everybody knows that the real thing that makes my chest bad is the weather!

Sometimes scientists find it very difficult to agree on whether something that 'everybody knows' is a real phenomenon or whether it is just something that a group of people have noticed. Studying the effects of the weather is also very difficult, as some of them may be delayed or may be related to how they affect other things known to cause COPD. For example, people think that wet and damp conditions make COPD worse, but it could also be that these weather conditions increase the number of cigarettes someone might smoke in a day. Some people also say that hot and clammy weather makes them feel worse.

One thing is certain, though. It is more common to get problems with your COPD in the winter months, and this is thought to be due to an increase in the number of infections such as the common cold around at this time. This why we recommend that people with COPD get vaccinated against the flu and pneumonia (see Chapter 9, *Living with COPD*).

I've heard somewhere that allergies make you more likely to suffer from COPD. Is this right?

This information comes from research carried out in Holland, which showed that people who develop COPD are likely to have raised levels of allergic antibody (IgE) in their blood or positive reactions to skin allergy tests (skin-prick tests). You can also have a test done in which you breathe in a substance (in very small amounts) known to cause narrowing of the airways. Depending on how much of this substance is needed to cause your airways to narrow, you can be classed as having *bronchial hyper-reactivity*. (We often use the term 'twitchy airways'!) All it really means is that your airways have a tendency to become narrow. The researchers in Holland thought this was an important factor in developing COPD – in fact, it became known as the Dutch Hypothesis. Bronchial hyper-reactivity is also found in people with asthma, which is probably why you have made the link with allergies. At the present time there is no specific allergic trigger for COPD, but it is known that bronchial hyper-reactivity is more common in people who smoke.

I thought asthma could lead to COPD. Have I got this wrong?

Provided asthma has been diagnosed and treated properly, it does not usually lead to COPD. But there are a small number of people in whom it has taken a while to diagnose asthma, or who have particularly severe asthma, in which it is not possible to reverse the poor functioning of the airways. (See Figure 1.2 and the accompanying text.) If 'occupational' asthma is not recognised until late, it can lead to permanent lung damage.

How do I know whether my disease is severe or not?

COPD can be classified as mild, moderate or severe according to the results of breathing tests (see the section on breathing tests in Chapter 3, *How is COPD diagnosed?*). You can also get a feeling about this by asking yourself questions such as, 'Can I go upstairs OK?' or 'Can I carry the shopping?' or 'Can I walk as far as my friends?' Sometimes people have such severe COPD that they cannot get out of their own home, but many others can manage all right provided they walk at a pace that suits them. Sometimes it is possible to improve your fitness by regular exercise (see Chapter 8, *Exercise and fitness*).

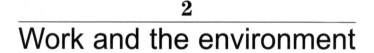

2
Work and the environment

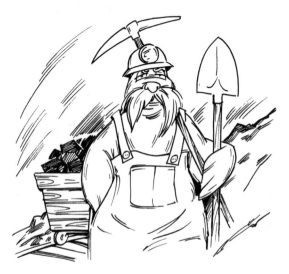

Occupation and lung disease

Workers are exposed to a wide variety of airborne contaminants on the job, such as dusts, welding fumes, gases and solvents. All have been associated with a variety of respiratory symptoms, including sneezing, coughing, chest tightness or difficulty breathing. There is now increasing concern that prolonged exposure over months or years can lead to long-term lung diseases such as chronic bronchitis, emphysema and asthma. Over the years a number of laws have been passed in an attempt to regulate exposure to these substances in the workplace.

How do I know if I might be in danger of developing respiratory conditions such as COPD at work?

It should be your employer's responsibility to inform you of potential hazards but you can also use your own senses. Here are some tips:

- Be aware of unusual eye irritation, especially when entering the work area. Some chemicals will irritate your eyes, nose and throat.
- Detecting an odour may indicate exposure to a dangerous amount of some workplace substances. You may smell a substance at first but after a while no longer notice it. This does not necessarily mean that your nose has become used to the odour, rather that it has temporarily lost its ability to detect the substance. Report odours to your manager.
- Visible clouds of dust or fumes usually mean that there is no ventilation system in the workplace, or that the existing system is not working well. Dust and fumes may irritate the nose, throat and lungs.
- Chemical spills can cause injuries and illnesses. Make sure that any chemicals are stored as recommended by the manufacturer. Spills should be cleaned up promptly and the reason for the spill investigated so that it doesn't happen again.

How can I find out whether I am at risk of developing COPD or having my COPD made worse by work?

Below are some questions that need to be considered.

- What am I working with?
- Is it a recognised cause or aggravating factor in COPD?
- How long after starting work did I notice any change in my breathing or having breathing difficulties?
- Do I notice any difference in my breathing when I am away from work?

Recurring chest symptoms such as persistent cough and shortness of breath or illnesses among workers may indicate a job-related health problem. If you notice a number of people in a work area frequently having the same symptoms or illnesses – especially if these conditions seem worse during working hours – they may be job-related.

Lots of people seem to get compensation for work-related asthma. What about COPD? How is it different?

Differences between asthma and COPD are discussed in Chapter 1 (*What is COPD?*). The major practical problem in diagnosing work-related COPD is that it is very difficult to distinguish between the effects of substances at work and the effects of cigarette smoking. It is common for people exposed to potentially damaging substances also to be smokers. This has not only made research in this area difficult but has also made it difficult for authorities to accept possible associations of substances at work with COPD.

Another problem is that people with asthma may not have received adequate treatment and go on to develop a more fixed breathing pattern, as opposed to the usual variable pattern. What this means is that people with asthma usually have symptoms that are reversible: if you feel bad one day, you may feel better the next (see the section 'Asthma and the others' in Chapter 1). Unfortunately, when the cause of asthma is related to the workplace, the symptoms might not vary so much and so affect people every day. Exposure at work can make this phenomenon more pronounced, leading to the opinion that the problem is work-related COPD when it may be work-related asthma. It is very important that you tell your doctor about breathing difficulties you have had throughout your life, as this may indicate that you have asthma as well as COPD.

I think that my work may be having an adverse effect on my breathing. Who is the best person to talk to?

If you work for a large organisation, it is likely that you will be able to see an occupational nurse or doctor. However, if this is not the case, it is best to make an appointment to see your own GP or practice nurse. There are a number of specialist centres for 'occupational lung disease' throughout the UK, if you feel you are not receiving a fair hearing, but it is customary for either your GP or a local specialist to check you out first.

I am a miner and have read a lot about mining causing emphysema. What has this got to do with COPD, and should I apply for compensation?

Emphysema is a condition in which the air sacs are damaged, and it is one of the many effects of long-term cigarette smoke on the lungs (see also Chapter 4, *Stopping smoking*). There has been a great deal of debate recently about the effects of coal mining on the lungs, and it is now agreed that exposure to coal dust can cause COPD. The effect is small but is independent of the effects of smoking (many coal miners are also smokers). It is now possible to receive compensation for the health effects of coal mining, and a number of chest specialists are part of a national panel set up to verify claims by miners. If you think that you might be eligible, you should contact your local union representative or speak to your GP or specialist. It is taking quite a long time to deal with the many miners seeking a review of their health but don't let that deter you.

I suffer from COPD but am pretty active. I am applying for a number of different factory jobs and have to fill out a health questionnaire on each occasion. I am concerned that if I put down COPD I won't get the job.

You should be pleased in many ways that your potential employer is concerned enough to want to find out about your health! These questionnaires are generally considered to be good practice. Provided that you are able to do the job as well as anyone else and are not putting yourself or other people in danger, there should be no problem in your being taken on.

There may be some examples of factory work that involve exposure to an agent known to cause breathing problems. In this instance, it may be part of the job specification (the 'job spec') that requires that there is no predisposing respiratory illness. You must remember that this is for your protection as much as anything else. There are, however, a few employers who do discriminate against people with respiratory and other chronic conditions. In this context, you might like to attach copy of a letter of support from your GP or specialist, but they are not obliged to provide you with this.

I went to see my doctor about breathing problems and he told me that I had COPD. He went on to ask me about my work as a welder and told me that my job may be making things worse. Could this be true, and might I lose my job?

In some ways you should be glad that your doctor is concerned about your health to this extent. There are some specialists who believe that welders who use cadmium may be more likely to develop emphysema-like changes in the lungs. This is especially true of people who also smoke. It is important that you explain as much as possible about what your job actually entails as opposed to just stating your occupation. It sounds as though you would benefit from evaluation by a specialist in work-related lung disease, and you should ask your GP to refer you on to them. Do not worry at this stage about losing your job; if your work *is* a problem, it is often possible for your employer to move you to a job where you are not exposed to the substance concerned.

I have spent a number of years working with asbestos. Will I get COPD?

Asbestos is not known to cause COPD but it can affect both the lungs and the lining of the lungs (the pleura). The majority of people do not suffer problems from working with asbestos but here are a few tips:

- Think about exactly when you worked with it. Who was your employer? How long were you working with them? What did your job actually involve? Did you wear any protective clothing or a facemask?
- Do you have any breathing problems now? If so, mention your exposure to asbestos to your GP.

- Are you in a trade union? If so, they may be able to offer you advice about any contact with asbestos you might have had.
- Remember that there is usually a gap of at least 10–15 years between your working with asbestos and developing any problems. But asbestos-related lung disease can appear over 50 years after your exposure, so it's always worth letting your doctor know about *all* the jobs you have done.

I am worried that a post-mortem will be done when I die because the doctors are concerned about the jobs I have undertaken. Please tell me this won't happen!

You must appreciate that everybody's situation is different and so we can't assure everyone that they will definitely not need a post-mortem examination. But there are some things we can say that might be helpful. As a general rule post-mortems are required to find things out that have not been known while people have been alive. So if it is known that you have lung disease related to your work, a post-mortem is not going to tell the doctors anything they don't already know! If you have COPD, it is extremely unlikely that a post-mortem is going to be required to find out whether your work was a factor in the disease. The only concern that doctors sometimes have is when there is a possibility that you have worked with asbestos.

Our advice would be to think carefully about all the jobs you have done and what you might have worked with and explain these to your doctor. Make a list, beginning with the date you left school, and then go through each job in turn – who you worked for, what you did and when you finished that job.

Atmospheric pollution

A pollutant is anything that contaminates the air, water, etc., with a harmful substance. A convenient way of categorising pollutants is to consider the indoor and outdoor environments. The most important *indoor* pollutant is cigarette smoke, and it is important to remember that you are affected not only by any cigarettes you smoke yourself but also by other people's cigarette smoke (so-called passive smoking). Most of the other indoor pollutants are important in connection with asthma, such as housedust mite and pet allergens but emissions from cooking and heating appliances can also have an effect on people with COPD. It is important to emphasise, however, that these effects are small and not thought to be important in the cause of COPD, only in making existing COPD worse. It is unlikely that you will be affected sufficiently to require changes to be made to your heating or cooking systems.

Outdoor pollutants are either natural or 'man-made' (vehicles or factories). The most common outdoor pollutant to cause respiratory symptoms is grass pollen, but this is not a significant factor in COPD. More important in COPD are the vehicle and industrial emissions – particularly sulphur dioxide (SO_2) that arises from the burning of coal, ozone from vehicle exhausts and the so-called particulate matter (explained below).

OZONE

Most people think that ozone is responsible for protecting us from the damaging effects of sunlight and that the increasing hole in the ozone layer in Earth's atmosphere is a bad thing. This is all true. But ozone can also be found at ground level and this is probably not such a good thing. At ground level ozone (O_3) is a highly reactive gas – that is, a form of oxygen that results primarily from the action of sunlight on hydrocarbons and nitrogen oxides emitted in fuel combustion. Exposure to ozone can produce significant airway narrowing and inflammation of the lung lining and respiratory discomfort, and is associated with hospital admissions and visits to accident and emergency (A&E) departments because of respiratory problems. The effects are more pronounced in people with asthma, and may be more severe in the summer. Some people think that ozone enhances the effect of grass pollen. There is currently little or no evidence linking exposure to ozone and COPD.

PARTICULATE MATTER

Particulate matter (PM) is a mixture of solid and liquid particles, and the majority of airborne particulate matter in the world's largest cities comes from diesel exhaust. If the particles are of a sufficiently small size (10 microns in diameter, to be precise!), they are easily inhaled and can damage the airways. Research has shown that raised levels of PM10 – particulate matter 10 microns or smaller – in the atmosphere have been associated with increased deaths and hospital admissions due to respiratory diseases, and also an increase in chest infections. It is unclear at present why this association has occurred, and the mechanism linking pollution episodes with respiratory disease is unknown. This means, in practice, that it is not possible to say that pollution 'causes' respiratory diseases, only that it is 'associated' with them.

SULPHUR DIOXIDE

Sulphur dioxide (SO_2) is formed when fuel containing sulphur (mainly coal and oil) is burned, and during metal smelting and other industrial processes. Following the fall of the Berlin Wall, a survey of breathing problems was undertaken in Leipzig, an East German industrial town with known high levels of sulphur dioxide. A significant increase in the symptoms of bronchitis was found there, and in similar industrial cities around the world. Again, it is difficult to be sure whether the effects of SO_2 on the airways and lungs make existing lung disease worse, or whether they are the cause of the problem. This is the subject of a good deal of research at the present time. Nevertheless, there is no doubt that avoidance of these substances is a good thing!

OXIDES OF NITROGEN

Oxides of nitrogen (NOX) form when fuel is burned at high temperatures. The principal sources of NOX are vehicles and fuel combustion. These oxides can irritate the lungs and lower resistance to respiratory infections such as influenza. Again, the majority of the effects are more pronounced in people with asthma, but the potential effect in people with COPD is currently being looked into.

So what does all this stuff about pollution mean? Should I be worried or not?

We're sorry to sound so uncertain but the situation is just not very clear-cut at the moment. The best take-home message we can come up with is that COPD is largely related to cigarette smoking and may also be associated with atmospheric pollution and work-related exposures – particularly to coal dust. More research is needed before we can accurately determine the role of pollution in COPD.

Aaargh! Everybody tells me to stop smoking but I know that if I didn't live in this city my lungs would be fine.

This is a common statement made by people who have COPD! Whilst it is possibly true to say that atmospheric pollutants can make people with COPD feel a good deal worse, the evidence that cigarette smoking causes COPD is overwhelming and you should make every attempt to stop smoking. Ways to do this are discussed in Chapter 4.

What is it about the weather that makes my COPD so bad?

This is a very difficult question to answer and we suspect that different people will be affected in different ways. Changes in the weather may affect people as a consequence of changes in temperature. This effect is particularly prominent with sudden bouts of cold or periods of very hot weather. Different climates may make it more or less possible for infectious agents – particularly viruses and bacteria – to thrive, and you may find that it's just that you're coming down with the same cold as everyone else.

I live in a large town and always cough up phlegm and wheeze during the day. I recently went on holiday to Spain and hardly had any breathing problems at all. Should I move to Spain?

Wouldn't it be lovely if moving one's possessions around the world were easy – we could just try out a number of different places for a while and see how we got on! Whilst it may be possible that you are affected in some way by living in the city, it is equally possible that you are not made worse by what you think is the problem. For example, when you spend time in another country you also spend time in another house. As people spend, on average, more than 90 per cent of their day indoors, you may be feeling better because of being away from a factor in the house as opposed to different air outside. Having said that, there are significantly lower levels of many atmospheric pollutants in coastal areas and these locations are also usually more breezy. It's therefore not wholly surprising that people find them a good place to be! But uprooting yourself – especially to another country – is a major undertaking, so be sure to consider all aspects of such a move before taking the plunge.

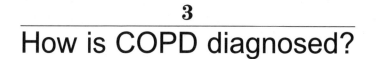

3
How is COPD diagnosed?

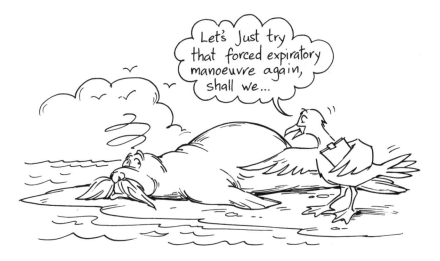

It is important to distinguish COPD from other sorts of lung disease so that you can be given the most appropriate treatment. You may have already read the section on symptoms in Chapter 1 (*What is COPD?*) but if you haven't, turn to it now to get an idea of the sort of symptoms that are associated with COPD. The main focus in this chapter is the use of lung function tests. Lung function tests are important in making a diagnosis of COPD and help give us information about how severe the disease is. Simple tests can be undertaken in many GP surgeries but patients are also referred to hospital to have tests done.

Spirometry

My GP is referring me to a clinic to have spirometry done. What is this?

COPD is usually accompanied by some degree of narrowing of the airways. This is often more pronounced when people are asked to breathe out as fast as they can. We can measure the degree of airway narrowing using a machine called a *spirometer* and the procedure undertaken is termed *spirometry* (see Figure 3.1).

There are a number of different types of spirometer – some of which are small enough to be held in your hand and others which are mounted on stands.

Before you do a spirometry test, an accurate measurement of your height will be made to allow any results to be compared with those from a 'normal' population. Usually you will be asked to sit down with, or in front of, the spirometer and take a few 'normal' breaths in and out. You then have to take as deep a breath in as possible before blowing out through the spirometer

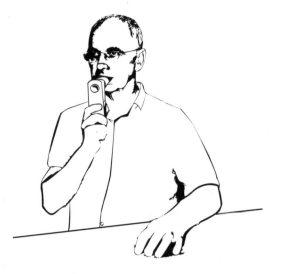

Figure 3.1 Performing spirometry

as hard and as fast as you can until you feel you have 'emptied' your lungs of air. We call this procedure a *forced expiratory manoeuvre.* It sometimes makes people feel a little dizzy, which is why you need to do it sitting down. We normally ask people to perform three tests, in order to check that we have their best result, or reading.

Spirometers have specially designed mouthpieces through which you must blow to give an accurate reading. People sometimes find this difficult so don't be surprised if the operator checks this aspect of your technique thoroughly to make sure that all the air you blow out goes into the spirometer and not outside the mouthpiece. Occasionally you can also 'lose' some air through your nose, and if we think this is going to be a problem we'll ask you to wear a nose-clip (a bit like a plastic clothes-peg) to prevent this.

When my GP told me that she wanted me to have a spirometry test, she talked about 'FEV-one' and 'FVC'. What are these?

Spirometry allows us to record two main results: FEV_1 and FVC.

FEV_1 stands for **F**orced **E**xpiratory **V**olume in 1 second, and measures how many litres of air you were able to blow out in the very first second of performing spirometry. It is the main measure used to identify any airway narrowing. The person measuring spirometry normally has access to a set of tables, which will allow them to compare your FEV_1 with a value known to be in the normal range. Usually, younger and taller males have larger lungs and will therefore have larger FEV_1 measurements, so these tables compare FEV_1 values depending on your age, height and sex. FEV_1 is measured in litres (L) and the value obtained from your efforts is compared with a suitable 'matching' population. This result is usually expressed as a percentage of predicted – '%Pred'.

FVC stands for **F**orced **V**ital **C**apacity, and is a measure of the total volume of air you were able to blow out through the spirometer. This too is measured in litres and can be expressed as a percentage of the predicted value for someone of your age, height and sex.

The spirometry operator talked about the FEV_1:FVC ratio. What is this?

When you do a spirometry test it is normal to blow out at least 75–80 per cent of your FVC in the first second – i.e. your FEV_1 should be 75–80 per cent of your FVC. Because the FEV_1 and FVC are known to have this relationship, it is usual to express their results in the form of a ratio as well as a percentage of the predicted value. Thus the normal FEV_1/FVC should be around 75–80 per cent. A value below this implies either a disproportionate decrease in FEV_1 or increase in FVC, both of which may occur in COPD.

Can these tests tell me how severe my COPD is?

Yes, they can. FEV_1 and FVC have been used to categorise COPD into mild, moderate and severe disease.

Mild COPD:	FEV_1 between 50 and 80% predicted
Moderate COPD:	FEV_1 between 30 and 49% predicted
Severe COPD:	FEV_1 less than 30% predicted

If I have moderate disease now, is there any chance I may be able to improve it to have only mild disease in the future?

As a general rule, your breathing tests will not improve very much. This is partly because of how COPD works and partly because it is normal for our lung function tests to get worse (decline) as we get older. It is possible to see some improvements with drug treatments (see Chapter 5, *Treatment*) or with exercise (see Chapter 8, *Exercise and fitness*).

Will I always have to perform spirometry whenever I go to see the doctor?

This depends a little on your doctor. Nearly everyone accepts that spirometry is essential for making a diagnosis of COPD but opinion differs as to whether regular measurements are as important in monitoring your disease as simply asking you how you are. If there seems to be any dramatic change in your breathing – whether better or worse – it is likely that you will be asked to repeat the spirometry. Many hospital specialists routinely ask their patients to perform spirometry when attending their clinics – sometimes even before you go in to see them.

I know about spirometry but not about the 'reversibility test', which a fellow patient was talking about. What is a reversibility test?

One of the differences between COPD and other types of airways disease is that the degree of airway narrowing does not change very much from day to day. This is in contrast to someone with asthma, in whom the degree of narrowing can change quite dramatically, either spontaneously or in response to certain treatments. It is therefore sometimes appropriate practice to perform spirometry before and after taking certain treatments to assess any change in your spirometry values. With some drugs (bronchodilators) this test may be done at only one visit but with others (steroids) you may need to take the treatment for some time before re-testing.

Do not worry if you have not had a reversibility test performed, as different health professionals attach different degrees of significance to the test. What is most important is whether a particular treatment makes you feel better.

What is a post-bronchodilator FEV$_1$? My husband's GP said he'll need to check this.

Many people with COPD have symptoms that can be helped by inhalers (see Chapter 6, *Inhalers and nebulisers*). The most commonly prescribed inhalers are called bronchodilators and, as their names suggest, they are designed to increase (dilate) airway (broncho) calibre. Measurement of spirometry following the use of such an inhaler is called post-bronchodilator FEV$_1$. Its importance lies in the fact that we use it to help decide something about the natural history of someone's COPD rather than to determine any specific treatment you require. Unfortunately, the lower your post-bronchodilator FEV_1, the worse your overall long-term outlook.

My GP forgets that I don't really understand the jargon she uses. What is a flow/volume curve or flow/volume loop?

When you blow into the spirometer as fast and as hard as you can, it is possible to record a characteristic pattern (or trace) on a chart. Indeed, many spirometers now print out these patterns for you to see, and the larger spirometers have a type of graph paper and pen specifically designed to generate these traces. It is possible to generate two types of graph when you perform spirometry – the volume/time curve and the flow/volume curve (sometimes called the flow/volume loop).

The **volume/time curve** measures the volume in litres on the vertical (y) axis and time in seconds on the horizontal (x) axis. It is from this curve that the measurements FEV_1 and FVC are calculated (see Figure 3.2a).

The **flow/volume loop** measures flow on the y axis (in litres per second or litres per minute) and volume (in litres) on the x axis (see Figure 3.2b).The significance of the flow/volume loop is that it can give an insight into what is happening in the smaller airways of the lungs.

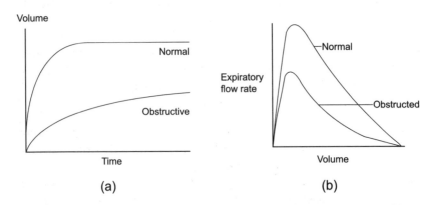

(a)   (b)

Figure 3.2 (a) An example of a volume/time curve.
(b) An example of a flow/volume loop.

Other lung function tests

What extra tests of lung function are performed at the hospital, and should everybody have them?

A large number of breathing tests may be performed in hospital breathing-test departments – or cardiorespiratory departments as they are usually called – but not all are relevant to people with COPD and not everyone needs to have them done. Broadly speaking, we are able to perform measurements of:

- lung volumes,
- gas exchange,
- oxygen and carbon dioxide (blood gas analysis).

Lung volumes When the airways are very narrowed or severely damaged, as can occur in COPD, it is sometimes not possible to breathe out all the air you take in. On breathing out your very small airways can collapse down, 'trapping' the gas in your air sacs. Over a long period of time this trapping can increase the total capacity or volume of your lungs and is in part responsible for some of the changes in the shape of the chest that some people with COPD experience. But before you ask yourself whether having 'larger' lung capacity may in fact be helpful, remember that the gas causing the increased capacity is 'trapped' and therefore useless. Indeed, it can often be a real hindrance, causing people to feel they cannot take an 'efficient' breath in. The techniques for measuring lung volumes vary between hospitals but often you will be asked to sit in a glass box called a body box. Some people may find this a little claustrophobic but the test rarely lasts more than 10–15 minutes.

Gas exchange The oxygen you breathe in has to get into your bloodstream in order to be useful to you. It does this by crossing over from your air sacs (alveoli) into a fine network of blood vessels (capillaries) in your lungs. At the same time as the oxygen enters your bloodstream, carbon dioxide leaves and enters your air sacs ready for you to breathe it out. This process is called *gas exchange* and is the primary function of your lungs. In some forms of COPD this process of gas exchange can be impaired and be responsible for your symptoms. It is possible for us to measure the efficiency of gas exchange in the cardiorespiratory department, but we usually reserve its use for people in whom the diagnosis of COPD is in doubt or for those who have symptoms out of proportion to the level of FEV_1 measured.

Blood gases If you have severe COPD (see the categories outlined a few questions earlier) there might be such a deficiency in the process of gas exchange that your levels of oxygen in the blood may be low. It is important to recognise this, because low oxygen levels can interfere with the performance of other organs in your body – in particular with the function of your heart. At present it is a good idea to think about having your blood gases checked if your FEV_1 is in the 'severe' range (less than 30% predicted). In addition, there are some other signs to look out for or questions to ask yourself – for example, 'Are my ankles swollen?' or 'Have my fingernails looked dusky or blue?' These may be signs that your heart is not receiving enough oxygen, so be sure to mention them to the health-care worker looking after you. If you have been admitted to hospital before as an emergency and have had a blood sample taken from your wrist or groin to test for oxygen, you may be feeling apprehensive about having your oxygen level checked. Do not worry! In the cardiorespiratory departments of most hospitals oxygen samples are measured by making a small (yes, small!) prick in the earlobe. This is called *capillary gas testing*, and is as accurate as other measurements of oxygen. An anaesthetic cream is applied to the earlobe to stop it hurting at all.

A friend with asthma does airway tests using something called a peak flow meter. Should I be given this too?

A peak flow meter measures *peak expiratory flow* (PEF), which is another measurement of airway calibre. The PEF meter is small and portable and can be prescribed on the NHS (see Figure 3.3). Peak expiratory flow is not as difficult to perform as spirometry but gives information only about narrowing of the larger

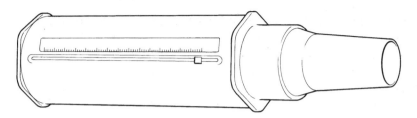

Figure 3.3 The Clement Clarke Standard Peak Flow Meter, which is one of the various types of peak flow meter available.

airways. Spirometry gives information about both large *and* medium-sized airways, which is thought to be of more use in diagnosing COPD.

The main reason why people with COPD are not usually given PEF meters is really that our experience suggests that the values very rarely change as they do in asthma and do not provide us with any more information than a one-off measurement of spirometry. However, some people with COPD are given PEF meters as part of trials of new drugs or in circumstances when their doctor or nurse may also wonder whether they have asthma as well as COPD (it is possible for the two conditions to occur together).

4
Stopping smoking

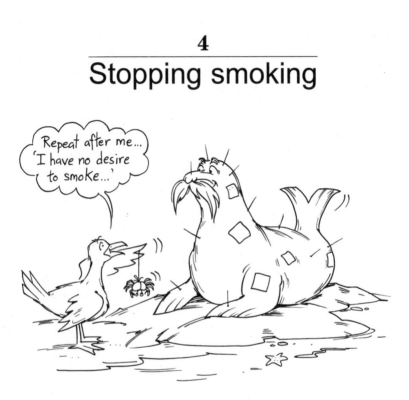

We are sure that the overwhelming majority of readers of this book realise how important it is to stop smoking. It is the best thing anyone can do for his or her health and there has never been a better time to stop for good. There are safe and effective treatments available both with and without a prescription, specialist NHS 'smoking cessation' clinics, and doctors and nurses are better equipped than ever to help you succeed. Yet many people feel they cannot ask their doctor for help, because they see their chest problem as self-inflicted, or are embarrassed about their smoking or are simply afraid of not succeeding.

Benefits of stopping smoking

Stopping smoking is the single most important thing you can do to prevent your COPD from getting worse. No matter how long you have smoked, you will notice a benefit. Within a year most people will be virtually free of cough and phlegm, and have less risk of chest infections. Medication will work more effectively. If you have mild COPD, stopping smoking might be the only treatment you need! It is vital to realise that, no matter how long you have smoked, it is never too late to stop. Table 4.1 outlines the progressively greater benefits you achieve the longer you stop smoking.

Table 4.1 Benefits of stopping smoking

Time since quitting	Benefits to health
20 minutes	Blood pressure and pulse return to normal
8 hours	Blood nicotine and carbon monoxide levels halved, oxygen levels normal
24 hours	Carbon monoxide eliminated from the body. Lungs start to clear of mucus/phlegm and other smoking debris
48 hours	No nicotine in the body. Ability to taste and smell greatly improved
72 hours	Breathing easier. Bronchial tubes begin to relax and energy levels increase
2–12 weeks	Circulation improves
3–9 months	Cough, wheeze and breathing problems improve. Lung function may improve by up to 10 per cent
1 year	Risk of heart attack falls to about half of that of a smoker
10 years	Risk of lung cancer falls to half that of a smoker
15 years	Risk of heart attack the same as someone who has never smoked

Why is it hard to stop smoking?

I have tried to stop smoking many times but can never manage more than a day; why?

Cigarettes contain nicotine, a substance as addictive as heroin and cocaine. Nicotine is a powerful stimulant that works directly on the pleasure centres of the brain by releasing 'feel-good' brain chemicals such as serotonin and dopamine: when you smoke, you feel good! Cigarettes are also highly efficient delivery systems, transporting nicotine in cigarette smoke via the lungs directly to the brain in about seven seconds: quicker than an intravenous injection. But stimulation of these pleasure centres is followed by 'rebound depression', as levels of the pleasure brain chemicals fall and others, such as noradrenaline, take over. This chemical is responsible for the unpleasant side-effects associated with craving. So you are prompted to light up another cigarette to relieve your craving, you feel good again, and so the cycle continues. That is why cigarette smoking is now recognised as an addiction, not just a habit, and why it can be so difficult to stop.

If nicotine is so addictive, why is it allowed in cigarettes?

Although nicotine is highly addictive and not without side-effects, it is a relatively less harmful constituent of tobacco smoke. Nicotine is known to constrict blood vessels and stimulate clotting of the blood in the capillaries, the smallest blood vessels. Cigarette smoke contains at least 4,000 chemicals – including arsenic, a well-known poison; formaldehyde, better known as preserving fluid; tar; and carbon monoxide. Of these chemicals, 600 are known to cause cancer; one of these is benzene. Every cigarette contains 190 micrograms (mcg or µg) of benzene, yet Perrier water was withdrawn from sale when it was found to contain only 4.7 micrograms per litre. When lit, a cigarette releases a cocktail of toxic gases and tar, and it is these substances that cause the most damage to our bodies.

How are the lungs harmed by cigarettes?

Although the way that cigarette smoke causes COPD is not yet fully understood, we do know the following. The lung damage caused by cigarettes includes excess production of sputum (phlegm) and the inability to clear it effectively, the build-up of scar tissue and the loss of elasticity in the lungs, and the destruction of lung tissue that disrupts the lung's ability to get oxygen into the blood and carbon dioxide out. Everybody responds differently to these effects, which is why someone in their early forties can develop severe COPD whilst others smoke heavily for years and do not develop breathing problems. We don't yet know why these differences exist.

Cigarette smoke contains tiny sparks heated to around 200°C (400°F), too small to see or feel, which are sucked into the air passages with each drag. These tiny sparks damage the tiny hairs (cilia) that line the airways by burning some away and paralysing many others so that they cannot function effectively. They are then replaced with fibrous scar tissue that reduces the elasticity of the airways, making it harder for them to expand. Imagine the scar tissue that a burn leaves behind: the skin becomes harder to the touch and more rigid – it loses its elasticity. The same thing happens in the airways of a smoker.

Tar and toxic chemicals damage the delicate linings of the air passages. In an effort to wash out tar and protect the lining, mucus-secreting glands in the airways increase in size and number and the production of phlegm increases. Stimulation of sensory nerve endings that become exposed in damaged airway linings leads to increased coughing, but the damage to the cilia makes it difficult to clear the excess phlegm (expectorate). This process, known as bronchitis, can lead to more frequent chest infections. Anyone who produces phlegm on most days for three consecutive months over a period of two years is said to have chronic bronchitis.

The body's immune system sends cells to the airways and the lungs; they release chemicals to neutralise the toxic chemicals from cigarette smoke. In some people this process leads to the breakdown and destruction of alveoli (where gas exchange normally takes place across a thin membrane). This condition is emphysema. When the alveoli are destroyed, the surface area for gas exchange is reduced and the body becomes deficient in oxygen. This process also adds to the loss of elasticity in the lungs.

Carbon monoxide in cigarette smoke makes it even more diffi-cult for the body to get enough oxygen. It, too, can cross the thin membrane of the alveoli, where it displaces oxygen in the blood. This is why breathing improves very quickly after stopping smoking. The result is poorer distribution of oxygen throughout the rest of the body.

King James I of England (VI of Scotland) wrote 400 years ago that tobacco smoke was

'Loathsome to the eye, hateful to the nose, harmful to the brain, dangerous to the lungs.'

He was right!

But isn't smoking just a habit?

Addiction to nicotine in cigarettes is the main reason why most people who smoke find it so hard to quit but obviously other factors are involved. The simple repetition of 10 to 12 puffs on 20 cigarettes a day produces 200–250 hand-to-mouth movements a day, nearly 100,000 per year; that is a powerful habit! Smoking is also associated with pleasurable everyday activity such as having a cup of coffee, or relaxing after a meal, and with social activities such as going to the pub. Many people who smoke believe that cigarettes make them feel relaxed and less stressed but the inabil-ity to smoke when in certain situations or environments leads to anxiety and actually increases stress levels. For many people smoking is 'part of who I am', 'all my friends smoke – I would feel left out if I stopped'; along with weight gain and fear of failure, these are powerful reasons for continuing to smoke.

So although smoking is a pleasurable experience, at some stage most people want to stop, for reasons such as health and finance. When they try, though, they realise that they have to cope not only with a habit but also with all the associations of their 'old friend'. It is the combination of habit, associated behav-iours and addiction that makes stopping smoking difficult.

**I am worried that if I stop smoking I will put on weight.
Will I, and what can I do to help myself?**

Smoking speeds up the body's metabolism so when you stop
smoking your metabolism and body weight will return to their
natural state. The weight gain from this should be no more than
7–10 pounds, a small amount, especially if you think about the
long-term benefits of stopping smoking to your lungs and general
health, and should not be too much of a deterrent.

However, we do not want to take the subject of weight too friv-
olously as fear of getting heavier can be a reason to continue
smoking. Your appetite may increase just because food will smell
and taste better! Below are our top tips for controlling your
weight and appetite, gleaned from people who have stopped
smoking themselves.

* It is probably best not to diet and stop smoking at the same
  time, but try not to suck sweets and eat fattening food in
  your attempt to overcome a craving for cigarettes.
* Eat regular meals to help you avoid snacking.
* If you do need a snack, stick to low-sugar sweets and keep
  a nibble box of non-fattening food nearby. Sticks of raw
  carrot and celery are good substitutes as they are crunchy
  and take time to chew. (Since he gave up smoking, JM's
  brother-in-law has never been without a pack of sugar-free
  mints!)
* Taking some form of exercise will benefit you in many
  ways, helping to keep your weight down, improving your
  general fitness and distracting you from your cravings.
  Quite a few people have told us that they have more
  energy, less cough and wheeze, and can walk further
  without getting short of breath.
* You may be able to access 'exercise on prescription'
  schemes where you can join classes at a local leisure
  centre for a reduced fee. Look out for information at your
  GP's surgery or the local leisure centre.

Can I just cut down?

Will switching to a low-tar or menthol cigarette be less harmful to me?

Unfortunately, no. Low-tar cigarettes are not really low tar. They contain the same amount of tar as ordinary cigarettes but are fitted with a denser filter. As it is nicotine that you are craving, you will tend to draw harder on the cigarette to get the equivalent high, thus cancelling out the effect of the filter. Menthol cigarettes contain the same amount of nicotine, tar and toxic chemicals as all other cigarettes; they just have a different flavour. The only way to reduce the risk of harm from cigarettes is to stop smoking for good.

What about cutting down the number of cigarettes I smoke, or switching to cigars or a pipe?

If you try to reduce the number of cigarettes you smoke, you will tend to take longer and deeper puffs of each cigarette and smoke it right down to the tip to satisfy your craving for nicotine. Although pipe and cigar smokers are not thought to inhale, cigarette smokers who switch generally do. Cigars in particular have a higher tar load than cigarettes, so you are actually increasing the amount of tar you inhale into your lungs. Although anything you do to reduce your exposure to cigarette smoke is to be applauded, it is only complete cessation that will produce improvements in your chest symptoms and prevent your condition from getting worse.

How to stop smoking

All right, I'm convinced that cigarettes are bad for me. But how can I stop smoking?

Your own motivation to stop is vital to your success, and having COPD is a powerful reason to stop smoking. Even if you have tried before, you now know that stopping is the one thing

that will improve your symptoms and prevent your condition
from getting worse.

You can assess your own level of motivation to quit by imag-
ining, on a scale of 1 to 10, how important it is for you to quit:
1 indicates not at all important and 10 indicates very important.
You can use the same method to assess your level of confidence to quit: 1 is that you are not at all confident that you can
quit and 10 is that you are very confident. You can then discuss
these levels with your GP or nurse, who can help you to sustain
or improve your motivation and confidence during the quit
attempt.

PREPARATION

Planning ahead is vital. Imagine you are fighting a war and that
each day is a battle you can win! Think about your past attempts
and why they were unsuccessful. You can learn from your past
experience and identify the reasons why you started smoking
again.

It may be useful to write down your thoughts so that you can
refer to them in the future.

- What is the longest time you have ever stayed stopped?
- What methods have you tried to help you stop?
- What helped?
- What didn't help?
- Did you find it difficult at particular times of the day or in
  certain situations?
- What made you start smoking again?

Don't be worried about past failures. Most people make a few
attempts before they manage to give up smoking for good. As
Mark Twain remarked:

'Giving up smoking is easy. I've done it hundreds of times.'

There are other things you can do that will increase your chances
of success.

- Keep a diary for a few days of the cigarettes you smoke. When did you smoke them, what were you doing, who were you with, how much did you need or enjoy each cigarette?
- Use the diary to identify the hard-to-give-up cigarettes and plan alternative activities for the times when you would normally smoke them.
- Identify family, friends or colleagues who can support you.
- Make a list of personal targets with a corresponding rewards list.
- Read motivational and information leaflets. Use star charts to mark off each day you are successful.
- Make a note of 'stop smoking' helplines, and use them if you are having a bad day.
- Quitting with another person can increase your chances of success.
- Set a quit day and stick to it!
- On quit day throw away all cigarettes, lighters and ashtrays.
- Save the money you would normally spend on cigarettes in a jar or separate account and reward yourself after a week or two. You will be amazed a how quickly it mounts up. Smoking 20 a day costs £30 week, £130 per month, £1,600 a year!

GET HELP

Perhaps the most important thing you can do to improve your chances of stopping smoking for good is to ask for help. Most GP practices and hospital clinics offer some form of 'smoking cessation' service or will be able to refer you to a specialist NHS clinic. Most of these clinics offer one-to-one or group sessions. Your local pharmacist may be another good person to talk to. We know from many research studies that you can double or treble your chances of stopping smoking by getting support and using medication, so ring your local surgery and find out what is on offer.

I am scared of stopping smoking. How will I feel?

Most people get some cravings and withdrawal symptoms when they stop smoking, which vary in frequency and intensity from person to person (see Table 4.2). Most of these last less than four weeks and can be relieved by using medication. Individual cravings are short lived and last only about three minutes. Try to distract yourself and the moment will pass. If you know what to expect, you can plan ahead and be better prepared when symptoms occur.

Table 4.2 Cravings and withdrawal symptoms

Withdrawal symptom	Duration
Light-headedness	Less than 48 hours
Night time awakening	Less than 1 week
Poor concentration	Less than 2 weeks
Craving	2 weeks or more
Irritability/aggression	Less than 4 weeks
Depression	Less than 4 weeks
Restlessness	Less than 4 weeks
Increased appetite	Approximately 10 weeks

Your desire to smoke will gradually subside after a few weeks and withdrawal symptoms and cravings will disappear. Hang on to the positive feelings of well-being you will have as you manage another smoke-free day and your lungs liberate themselves of carbon monoxide, tar and nicotine. If you have a bad day, remember why you want to stop smoking. Think about how positive you feel when you don't smoke and the benefits you will see in the future. Use a 'stop smoking' helpline, such as Quit, for support.

How will I know if I need to use medication to help me stop smoking?

Most people who smoke do not continue to do so out of choice, but because they are addicted to nicotine. Nicotine replacement therapy (NRT) is available on general sale and on prescription. The 'stop smoking' tablet bupropion (Zyban) is available only on prescription. Both of these treatments are much more effective if combined with ongoing support. Your nurse, doctor or pharmacist will be able to advise you on the most appropriate medication for you. As a rule, if you smoke more than 20 a day or have your first cigarette of the day within 30 minutes of waking, you are more likely to benefit from medication to help you quit. But if you are struggling to stop, especially if you have cravings no matter how many you smoke, ask for help.

Nicotine replacement therapy

How does nicotine replacement therapy work?

Nicotine replacement therapy (NRT) provides lower levels of nicotine, which are delivered more slowly than with cigarette smoking, and without the tar and toxic gases. This will reduce your cravings and withdrawal symptoms and should allow you to concentrate on breaking your smoking habits. This normally takes 8–12 weeks, so you should think of NRT as a course of treatment. Most people find that higher doses are needed for 6–8 weeks and then the dose can be reduced over 2–4 weeks. NRT is not a replacement for cigarettes and you will not get the same kick – you will still need motivation and willpower.

All NRT is available on general sale in pharmacies and supermarkets but it is also sometimes available on prescription. Because NRT works best if you combine its use with ongoing support, we would advise you to make an appointment with your GP or practice nurse to discuss the options and see what services are available. If your GP prescribes NRT for you, he or she will want you to commit to not smoking and probably to attend every couple of weeks for up to three months to see how things are going and to give you further advice and support. Using NRT can double your chances of quitting.

There are lots of types of nicotine replacement. How do I know which one to use?

All NRT products work in the same way and are equally effective. In the end what you use will be down to personal choice. There are six types available:

- patches,
- gum,
- nasal spray,
- inhalator,
- microtablets,
- lozenges.

If you don't like chewing gum, gum is obviously not suitable for you; likewise if your skin is easily irritated, patches may not be appropriate. If you match the product to your personal taste, it is likely to be the best one for you.

Nicotine patches are very easy to use. You apply them to dry, non-hairy skin on your trunk or upper arm. You should change to a different site each day. They are available in formulations designed to last for 24 or 16 hours and in three strengths. The 24-hour patch may prevent the urge to smoke first thing in the morning but can cause sleep disturbance. The adhesive in all patches may cause skin irritation.

Nicotine gum is available in two strengths and a variety of flavours. Nicotine gum is used very differently from ordinary chewing gum. It should be chewed until you taste the flavour and then parked between your cheek and gum; this area of your mouth has a good blood supply, which picks up the nicotine from the gum. When you feel the desire to smoke again you chew for a few more moments, then park the gum again and continue this cycle. Each piece of gum lasts about 20–30 minutes and you can use up to 15 pieces in 24 hours, as you feel the need – on demand. If you chew continually, the gum tastes unpleasant and will not be as effective. Because you can use gum on demand, you can regulate the dose to your own needs. It may not be suitable if you wear dentures.

Nicotine spray produces higher peaks of nicotine than other forms of NRT, but still considerably lower than from cigarettes. The nicotine is sprayed into the nostril but shouldn't be sniffed up. It is used on demand when the urge to smoke occurs, to a

maximum of 64 sprays a day. The spray gives fast relief of cravings, and it is quite easy to adjust the dose to your personal
needs. It may cause irritation of the nose at first, but this
usually settles; however, some people cannot tolerate this side-
effect.

Nicotine inhalator is used with nicotine-impregnated cartridges. You inhale when the urge to smoke occurs until the
desire goes away. Each cartridge lasts for about 20 minutes of
intensive use, and most people will need to use between 6 and the
maximum of 12 cartridges a day. The inhalator will keep your
hands busy, and it is easy to regulate the dose.

Nicotine microtablets are placed under the tongue to dissolve
when the urge to smoke is felt. You can use one or two an hour
as needed, up to a maximum of 40 a day. They are easy to use and
discreet but they must be used correctly as they are wasted if
swallowed. Microtablets sometimes irritate the mouth but you
can prevent this by placing them in a different place under the
tongue each time you use one.

Nicotine lozenges are available in two strengths: 2mg and 4mg.
They dissolve slowly in the mouth over about 30 minutes. They
should be moved from side to side periodically. You can use one
or two an hour when you feel the urge to smoke, to a maximum
of 15 a day. Like microtablets, they are discreet and easy to use
but can cause throat irritation and indigestion.

I tried patches last time I tried stopping; why didn't they work?

All forms of NRT can double your chances of stopping smoking
but not every quit attempt is successful. Common reasons for
NRT not working include:

- stopping the NRT too soon,
- not using a high enough dose,
- continuing to smoke.

Some people stop their NRT or try not to use it because they worry about side-effects. We know that the list of possible side-effects on packs of NRT can look daunting but remember that they are the same as some of the side-effects from smoking! The risks from using NRT, though, are considerably less than those of continuing to smoke, and by using NRT as recommended you double your chances of stopping smoking.

In our experience, once someone has tried a form of NRT that did not work for them, they lose confidence in it. So it would probably be a good idea to discuss all the different forms of NRT with your doctor, nurse or pharmacist so that an appropriate alternative can be found. It is also important to remember that all medical treatment for stopping smoking is most effective with ongoing support, so ask to be referred to a 'smoking cessation' clinic.

The most important thing is not to be disheartened. Most people have more than one attempt at stopping smoking before they stop for good, so keep trying!

My doctor suggested that I use both a patch and an inhalator. Can I do this?

Although the makers of NRT products do not have a licence for combining different types, many doctors and specialist clinics do recommend this method, and there has been some research to suggest that it can be effective. It is less harmful to wear a patch and use an inhalator than to use a patch and smoke! So long as you have had medical advice to do this, there should not be any problems.

My mum is trying to stop smoking using a patch but is still having a few cigarettes every day. Is this dangerous?

It is not recommended to smoke and use NRT at the same time. We know some people who are coping really well, have a bad day, take their patch off, have a cigarette then put the patch back on again! Your mum should be congratulated for doing so well but the problem with continuing to smoke even a very few cigarettes is that she probably has not made the mental change to being a non-smoker. Honesty is the best policy. Your mum should have a chat with her doctor or nurse about her need for a cigarette so that an alternative strategy can be found. A specialist service may be able to help her move forward in her attempt to give up on cig-arettes for good. Try not to nag your mum, as she may resort to smoking in secret – she will benefit most from your support and understanding.

I bought some nicotine replacement therapy but the leaflet inside said it could be dangerous. Is it?

That leaflet is frightening, isn't it, but how would you feel if the same leaflet were inside your cigarette packet? The potential side-effects of NRT are exactly the same as the side-effects of continued smoking, but the risks of using NRT are considerably less. The next time you buy paracetamol look at the list of poten-tial side-effects. Will it stop you taking it the next time you have a headache?

The makers of NRT are playing on an uneven field. NRT is sold as a medicine, cigarettes are not. Don't use that list of potential side-effects as another excuse to carry on smoking. NRT is safe to use if you have COPD, but have a chat with your GP or practice nurse about its suitability for you.

After being a smoker for 30 years I managed to stop smoking using gum and patches six months ago, but still get cravings if I go out with my friends to the pub. What can I do?

Congratulations! It takes a lot of motivation and effort to stop smoking even with medication. Many people continue to get the odd craving even years down the line but it is vital that you resist. If you ask a relapsed smoker what made him or her start again they'll probably say that they just took a cigarette. Most people who start smoking again after quitting do so at times of stress or in a social situation when they are relaxed, so you are not on your own in finding going to the pub difficult.

We have found that people have different ways of dealing with these odd cravings. Remember that 'serious' cravings last for a short period of time and if you can distract yourself the moment will pass. A patient of mine [JM] used to have a game of darts or pool and if all else failed he sat in the gents' toilets for five minutes! If you are finding it really hard, you could try using an on-demand NRT product such as an inhalator just when you are out, but remember this is giving you nicotine that you are no longer used to having, so you may find that you dislike the taste or you may even feel a bit sick or light-headed. Your doctor and nurse will want to help you stop smoking for good, so if you need extra help, ask for it. In the end, do anything you can (within reason!) to resist taking a cigarette.

Bupropion (Zyban)

I have heard that there is a drug to help you stop smoking. What is it and how does it work?

This drug is called bupropion, also known as Zyban (the brand name given by its manufacturer). It works directly on the addictive pathways in the brain and helps to prevent cravings and withdrawal symptoms rather than reduce cravings by replacing nicotine the way NRT does. It can be very effective although, like NRT, it does not replace motivation and willpower and works best when combined with ongoing follow-up and support. One research study has shown that it is safe and effective in helping people with COPD to stop smoking. Over all, it has some of the best quit rates in comparison with other smoking cessation methods, and has been endorsed for use by the UK's Institute for Clinical Excellence (NICE) as a safe and effective treatment for helping people to stop smoking. It is a prescription-only medication and cannot be bought over the counter like NRT.

It is usually prescribed as one tablet a day for the first seven days then twice a day with at least 8 hours between doses for an overall 8-week course. You would be asked to stop smoking 10–14 days into the course but to continue taking Zyban for the full 8 weeks. If you had not managed to stop smoking by the end of the 8-week course, it is unlikely that bupropion would work for you this time. The reasons for this can be complex: it may be that your motivation to quit was not as high as it could be or that this was just not the right time. Bupropion might work if you have another attempt but you should discuss this with your doctor.

We have found that about 70–80 per cent of people who take bupropion manage to stop smoking for at least a month, but some relapse and the overall quit rate at a year is about 30 per cent. However, the reasons for relapse are complicated. Cravings do not get worse after stopping bupropion, so willpower and your motivation to stay stopped are vital.

My father has been prescribed Zyban tablets by his GP. I don't want him to take them as I read in the paper that they are dangerous. Are they?

It can be very worrying when newspapers report problems with drugs, especially when you or a member of your family is taking that treatment. When Zyban (the brand name for the drug bupropion) was first introduced in the UK there were a few highly publicised deaths associated with its use, but on investigation the link between these deaths and Zyban was disputed. Most of the people who died had underlying smoking-related conditions (such as heart problems) and others were not taking Zyban at the time of their death. Others had circumstances or illnesses that were 'contraindications' to the use of Zyban but they had not told their doctor about them.

Bupropion (Zyban) is not suitable for everyone and doctors are advised not to prescribe it for people with certain conditions. Your father's doctor will have taken a detailed history from your father and checked that Zyban is safe for him. We have found that Zyban is generally well tolerated, and the most common side-effect is a dry mouth. Recognised side-effects of Zyban include sleeplessness, agitation, nausea and a rash. If your father experiences any of these symptoms, he should see his doctor for advice. Symptoms such as sleeplessness and agitation could be a sign of nicotine withdrawal.

The risks of continued smoking far outweigh the risks of using Zyban and it has helped millions of people world-wide to stop. It is a frightening fact that 300 people die every day from a smoking-related illness – that is one in two life-long smokers! Stopping smoking is very difficult, only 1–2 per cent of smokers manage to stop without help each year, and we have found that Zyban, pre-scribed with care to suitable people, is a very useful weapon in the fight against nicotine addiction.

Other methods

My GP says I am not able to have any medication to help me give up smoking. What can I do?

Medication may not be suitable for everyone yet many people still manage to stop smoking, and you have an important personal reason to succeed. Even if drug treatment is not appropriate for you, you should still ask your GP or practice nurse for advice and support as this can increase your chances of success. Quitting with another person can also help, as you can support each other along the way. Some specialist services may offer alternative therapies such as relaxation, acupuncture or hypnotherapy that may be of benefit to you.

Will complementary therapy such as hypnotherapy or acupuncture help me stop smoking?

Although we can offer you little or no scientific evidence that hypnotherapy and acupuncture are effective smoking cessation therapies, we know a few people who state that these methods were highly effective for them. The idea of treating you as a whole person, rather than someone who has COPD or is trying to stop smoking, is an important part of any complementary therapy; this is a view we strongly support.

Hypnosis in particular may help by improving relaxation and reducing stress, leaving you better able to cope with cravings. Our main advice is to seek a qualified, registered practitioner (contact details of the British Medical Acupuncture Society and the British Hypnotherapy Association are in the Appendix, *Useful addresses*). Some NHS specialist smoking cessation clinics offer these therapies, usually free of charge. Contact your local smoking cessation service to find out what is available. You should be able to find the number in the telephone directory, your library or from your GP's surgery.

5
Treatment

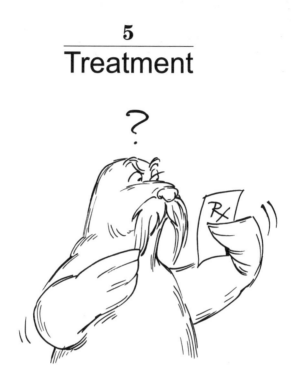

This chapter deals with the main medical treatments for COPD available in the UK. Non-drug treatments and oxygen therapy are dealt with in more detail in Chapters 6 and 7.

There are many different drugs available for use in COPD but not everyone is on every treatment. If your own treatment is not named in this book, it does not necessarily mean that you are on the 'wrong' drugs; it is more likely that we have not had enough space in this book to mention every drug available. An added problem is that each drug has a minimum of two names. The *generic name* is the basic drug name, but each drug also has a *brand* (or *trade*) *name*, given by the manufacturer. For example, a commonly prescribed drug for reducing symptoms in COPD is salbutamol (generic name). This is best known by the brand name Ventolin, used by the leading manufacturer, but also has the name Aerolin when produced by a different company.

At the present time the only way to prevent COPD from getting worse is to give up smoking. People with very severe disease can be given oxygen (see Chapters 4 and 7 for more details) but this won't improve the airflow obstruction. Drug treatments used in COPD are aimed at performing three major tasks:

- reducing symptoms on a day-to-day basis,
- reducing flare-ups of COPD (exacerbations),
- making people feel better in themselves (sometimes referred to as 'improving quality of life').

Nearly all the treatments now used in COPD were initially developed for use in people with asthma. It is customary in asthma to classify drugs as those that try to prevent the disease ('preventers') and those that try to reduce the symptoms ('relievers'). Whilst this is not the case in COPD, you may still find that your treatments are grouped in this way to help you in working out which ones should be taken regularly, regardless of how well you are feeling, and which can be taken in varying amounts depending on how you are feeling. *Preventer* medications usually mean steroid-containing inhalers and *relievers* those not containing any steroids.

Inhaler drugs

The doctor has given me inhalers to help my COPD. How often should I use them?

This is a commonly asked question and, in many ways, the most important to establish. COPD symptoms do not tend to vary that much from day to day unless you are about to experience a flare-up of your condition, so it is likely that you will need to use the inhalers regularly. This is particularly important if you are prescribed a steroid inhaler, because you have to use it regularly to benefit from it. Most non-steroid inhalers are prescribed to allow you to vary the dose depending on how you feel – you may be told to use them 'as necessary' or 'as required'. There is one group of non-steroid inhalers, called long-acting bronchodilators, which should also be used regularly. Salmeterol (trade name Serevent), eformoterol fumarate (trade name Oxis) and tiotropium (trade name Spiriva) are three examples of this group.

As a general rule you should ask for written information about any treatment you are given, so that you can remind yourself how often you need to use it.

What is a bronchodilator? My uncle says that he uses this.

This group of drugs has been developed to relieve symptoms due to airway tightening or narrowing. Most bronchodilators are in the form of inhalers; some are available as tablets but very few people take these. Many of the bronchodilator preparations act within 15–20 minutes of inhalation but their effects last for only 4–6 hours. These are known as short-acting bronchodilators. In COPD there are two groups of inhaled short-acting bronchodilators – the beta-agonists and the anticholinergics. These are named after the ways in which the drugs are thought to work on the airways:

- beta-agonists cause the muscles in the airways to relax, which can make the airways wider and thus help breathing;
- anticholinergics can also do this but to a lesser degree; however, they can decrease the amount of mucus and phlegm you make, and this often makes people feel better.

Examples of beta-agonists are salbutamol (Ventolin) and terbutaline (Bricanyl), whilst ipratropium (Atrovent) is the most commonly prescribed anticholinergic inhaler. Combination preparations of beta-agonist and anticholinergic medications are also available, of which the brand name drug Combivent is the most commonly used.

Short-acting bronchodilators are often needed regularly but are often prescribed in a way that allows you to use them in larger doses if you are not feeling so well.

However, if you are using more short-acting bronchodilator than normal, or the effects are not lasting the usual 4–6 hours, your COPD is not well controlled and you should seek medical help.

Some bronchodilator drugs work for longer than six hours and are known as long-acting bronchodilators. These can also be either the beta-agonist type (salmeterol or eformoterol are examples) or the anticholinergic type (tiotropium is an example). These inhalers are prescribed for regular use, and should be considered as complementary to short-acting drugs rather than instead of these medications. A tablet form of the bronchodilator aminophylline (e.g. Phyllocontin), which is neither a beta-agonist nor an anticholinergic, is also available and can help some people with COPD. As a general rule, however, it is best to try to control the disease with inhalers, because they are associated with fewer side-effects.

My medication has recently been combined into one inhaler. Will it still work as well?

Combinations of various different types of medication for COPD have been available for some time and have largely been used by people with severe disease to reduce the total number of puffs they have to take. In all instances the individual drugs have been tested to show that they work at least as well as the individual treatments taken on their own. You may find this a more convenient way to use your medication and it may also reduce your prescription costs.

I have recently had my inhalers changed because of global warming! What is that all about?

If you have been taking an aerosol inhaler (see the section on inhalers in Chapter 6), you may have been issued with a change in device. Until recently, aerosol inhalers contained chlorofluorocarbons (CFCs). Some inhalers now contain alternatives to CFCs and have been developed in response to the need to protect Earth's atmosphere. Some of the newer inhalers feel and taste different but they contain the same type of treatment that you have used before.

A friend uses a steroid inhaler, which he finds really helpful. Why have I not been given this, too?

Steroid inhalers were initially developed for the treatment of asthma. They are the front-line inhalers for the prevention of asthma symptoms and are used early on in that disease. Things are different in COPD and we are still not yet certain which patients are most likely to benefit from steroid inhalers. Sometimes your doctor will test whether you need a steroid inhaler by giving you a course of steroid tablets (usually for two weeks) to see if you feel better. This 'steroid trial' isn't really supposed to be part of the assessment of COPD but has been thought to help in ruling out COPD from people who might have asthma, and may be something your doctor wishes to try. If, however, you have moderate to severe disease, it is increasingly likely that you will be asked to take a steroid inhaler regularly in an attempt to prevent flare-ups of your condition. Sometimes steroid is combined with your long-acting bronchodilator in the same inhaler; Seretide and Symbicort are examples of these combination inhalers.

If you are unsure why you are being asked to take any medication, do ask for clarification. It is well known that people are more comfortable taking treatment if they are settled in their own mind about what it is supposed to be doing!

I have two different inhalers. Does it matter which I take first?

If you are prescribed more than one inhaler, it is usually considered 'standard practice' to use a short-acting bronchodilator first and any other inhaler afterwards. It doesn't really make any difference, so our advice would be to do what works best for you. The most important thing is to take everything you are supposed to take!

If I forget to take a 'regular use' inhaler on one day should I take twice the amount on the following day?

It is quite common for people to forget the odd puff of medication here and there – particularly if you are feeling pretty well. It is also true, however, that regular use of treatment may be the reason you are feeling so well! Treatment that is prescribed for regular use – particularly inhaled steroids – takes some time to exert its effect, so missing an occasional dose will not matter. Hence there is no need to double up on the following day. However, regular use really does mean 'regular use'!

Steroids

What is prednisolone for?

Prednisolone is the most commonly prescribed steroid tablet in COPD. Its primary role is in the treatment of flare-ups of your condition. Flare-ups, or exacerbations, of COPD are often associated with inflammation of the airways because they have become infected. Prednisolone dampens down this inflammation and reduces the period of time your exacerbation lasts. It is not uncommon for you to be asked to take 6 or 8 steroid tablets every day for up to two weeks. This is often referred to as a 'course of steroids'. If you are unable to take tablets, prednisolone is also available in a soluble form, available as a brand name drug called Prednesol.

Sometimes you will be asked to take steroid tablets as part of a test to see whether a steroid-containing inhaler would be suitable for you to use regularly. The number of tablets and the duration of treatment are likely to be the same – 6 or 8 tablets every day for up to two weeks. This 'steroid trial' is not encouraged nowadays but your doctor might try it to check that you do not have asthma. Although it is a rare occurrence, a small number of people with COPD need steroid tablets every day. If you know someone who is taking steroid tablets regularly, please do not assume that this is the general rule. Your doctor will be committed to reducing to a minimum the number of steroid tablets you need to take, and the overwhelming majority of people do not require regular steroid tablets.

I'm worried about taking steroids. Aren't they harmful?

It is important to distinguish between different types of steroid and the different ways in which they are used. For example, the

steroids used to treat flare-ups of COPD are very different from
those used by body builders. They use anabolic steroids, whereas
we use corticosteroids. Corticosteroids have become a very important part of treating diseases of the lungs. Most people only need
steroids via an inhaler, and this has the advantage that the amount
required to achieve a desired effect is very low. The amount of cor-
ticosteroid used in a 'course of steroids' (see the previous answer)
is certainly greater than that used in an inhaler but there are no
long-lasting effects of using steroid tablets for two weeks.

Corticosteroids usually only cause problems in the small
number of people who require long-term treatment with steroid
tablets – for periods of months or years. In this instance side-
effects include weight gain, thinning of the skin, increase in blood
pressure, thinning of the bones (osteoporosis) and an increased
tendency to develop diabetes. None of these problems is
common, but all are recognised. This is why it is important to use
inhaled forms of steroid treatment wherever possible.

**I understand that the steroids used for COPD are safe
when used properly, but don't inhaled steroids have side-
effects too?**

When taken in low doses the only problem of inhaled cortico-
steroid therapy is hoarseness of the voice. This is greatly
improved by rinsing out your mouth after using your inhaler.
Some people use their inhaler just before brushing their teeth.

However, if higher doses of inhaled steroids are used, more
'local' problems are encountered, the most significant of which is
a fungal infection of the throat, known as oral candidiasis. This is
usually associated with a red rash and white spots at the back of
the throat. It often irritates the voice and can make the throat sore.
It is easy to treat and can often be prevented by using a different
device or a spacer (see the section on inhalers in Chapter 6).

At very high doses of inhaled steroids there have been reports
of thinning of the bones and also of cataracts and glaucoma.
Remember, though, that it is very rare for someone with COPD to
require such high doses and, in such a situation, the doctor will
keep a watchful eye on the patient.

Exacerbations and flare-ups

What is an exacerbation of my COPD?

An 'exacerbation' is the medical term used to describe deterioration in COPD, usually as a consequence of getting a chest infection. The sorts of things to look out for are an increase in breathlessness, an increase in the amount of phlegm you cough up or a change in colour of the phlegm if it is usual for you to cough it up. These symptoms should prompt you to seek medical attention, because you are likely to require antibiotics, and possibly even steroid tablets for a short time.

During a recent flare-up I noticed a bit of blood in my phlegm. Should I worry about this?

Whilst it is not uncommon for an infection to irritate the airways sufficiently to make you cough up red-stained phlegm, you should always mention this to your doctor. It is likely that you will need a chest x-ray to assess your lungs further and find out the cause.

Worries about treatment

I am worried about becoming 'addicted' to my treatment and needing ever-bigger doses. Can you reassure me?

This is a common concern of people who take any type of treatment regularly. There is no need to worry about your medication becoming less effective as time goes on. It is more likely that the nature of your COPD will change, and this may require a change in your treatment. An addiction is really a situation where your body feels unable to manage without a specific stimulus or treatment. If you are, or have been, a smoker, you may well remember that feeling!

Even if I don't become addicted to my regular treatment, can't I become resistant to all the antibiotics I am receiving?

Whilst it is possible to get infections that are resistant to some antibiotics, it is rare for these to cause long-term problems to people with COPD. The important issue is really how often you feel you need antibiotics, as there are other chest conditions that can seem similar to COPD but are in fact quite different. In practice, your doctor is likely to request a chest x-ray if you are getting lots of infections or in an instance where the antibiotics you took didn't seem to do their job. It is also possible, if appropriate, to send a sample of your phlegm to the laboratory to check it out for infection and to make sure that a particular antibiotic will work if prescribed.

Other treatments

There's a notice at my GP surgery that recommends annual vaccination against flu. Should I get these 'flu jabs'?

Yes, you should. These are an important part of preventing flare-ups of your COPD. Every year you should attend your surgery for a flu jab and about once every five years you should also receive an anti-pneumonia vaccination (brand name Pneumovax).

I tend to cough up a lot of sticky phlegm. Is there anything I can take to ease this?

Your doctor might consider something called mucolytic therapy, in which you take a drug that makes phlegm less sticky. *N*-Acetyl cysteine is designed to reduce the *viscosity* – the 'stickiness' – of phlegm. It is a fairly new treatment that may be helpful for people with chronic bronchitis and a recent analysis supports its use in COPD. There are currently two products now available on NHS prescription: carbocisteine and mecysteine. They seem to be particularly useful if you have moderate or severe COPD and are having trouble with sticky phlegm.

I know my disease is severe and the doctors have told me things won't get better. Isn't there anything I can try to help my breathing? I get so breathless.

It is a terrible feeling being breathless all the time isn't it. It is quite possible that your doctor may have prescribed oxygen for you by now, but if you want any more information about that, go straight to Chapter 7 (*Oxygen therapy*). Some people have tried drug treatments specifically for the relief of breathlessness, but they do not seem to suit everybody. Small doses of diazepam (Valium) or small doses of morphine help some people because they slow down the speed of your breathing.

It might be a good idea for you to ask your doctor if you can speak to a Macmillan nurse. We know that Macmillan nurses usually see people who have cancer, but some have quite a lot of experience in managing people with severe breathlessness and in some parts of the UK the Macmillan service is able to help very breathless people who do not have cancer. It may be worth a try.

6

Inhalers and nebulisers

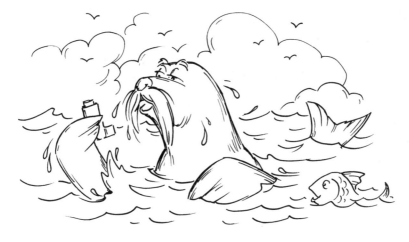

The ever-growing range of inhaler devices available for delivering your treatment can be overwhelming. This chapter describes each device in turn, how it works, how to use it and how it should be cared for. You will also find the answers to some of the most frequently asked questions about inhaler devices. The need for and use of nebulisers is dealt with in a separate section in this chapter.

Inhaler devices

The important thing to know about inhaler devices is that you have to use them correctly to ensure that you get the drug to where it is needed. Although this may sound obvious, many people use their inhalers incorrectly and are therefore not getting the benefit of the treatment. You should always be instructed how to use your inhaler by someone who has been trained in its use – for example, your doctor, nurse, pharmacist or physiotherapist. They should also check your inhaler technique at follow-up appointments to identify any problems or bad habits that have developed!

Why do I have to use an inhaler?

Using inhaled therapy rather than tablets may seem more trouble than it is worth, especially if you have found it difficult to perfect the correct technique, but the benefits should outweigh any problems. Inhaled therapy is delivered direct to the site where it is needed – your lungs. This direct delivery means that a smaller dose can be used than that given by a tablet, that the treatment will work faster, and that side-effects are minimised.

What inhalers are available?

There is quite a range of inhaler devices available for the treatment of COPD and other conditions such as asthma, and you will find illustrations of all of them in this chapter. There are three main types of inhaler:

- pressurised metered-dose inhalers (MDIs),
- breath-actuated inhalers (BAIs) – e.g. Autohaler and Easi-Breathe,
- dry powder inhalers (DPIs) – e.g. Accuhaler, Aerohaler, Clickhaler, Diskhaler, HandiHaler, Turbohaler.

Spacer devices are used with MDIs to increase the amount of drug deposited in the lungs, to reduce side-effects in the mouth and throat, and to overcome the problems of co-ordination inherent in MDIs used alone; for example, Able Spacer, AeroChamber, Nebuhaler, Volumatic.

All devices deliver a set dose of drug in each puff and are as effective as each other when used correctly. It is important, however, to select the right device for each individual, as the wrong choice of device can be the reason behind a lack of control of symptoms. Your doctor or nurse should help you to choose the most suitable device for you: they have to take into account the type of drug you need and which device provides it, whether you can use it correctly and whether it meets your individual needs. All inhaler devices come with an instruction leaflet that should be studied carefully before use.

What is a pressurised metered-dose inhaler?

The pressurised metered-dose inhaler (MDI) is the most commonly used inhaler device (Figure 6.1). Nevertheless, a lot of people find the technique difficult and a number of surveys have revealed that many of those using MDIs use them incorrectly. The main problem is that you need to co-ordinate breathing in the drug and pressing down on the canister with your finger. This is difficult to achieve, and even with careful practice many people (even doctors and nurses!) find it impossible. So it is vital that you have the opportunity to demonstrate and discuss your device technique with your doctor, nurse or pharmacist. If you cannot get the technique right, do not be disheartened. You can try adding a spacer device or switching to a breath-actuated or dry powder device.

MDIs should be stored away from extremes of temperature. The mouthpiece cover should always be replaced after use, to prevent dirt and particles from accumulating in the mouthpiece, which you could then breathe in the next time you use it. If the mouthpiece gets dirty, it can be wiped clean with a damp cloth. When MDIs are empty, they should be replaced by getting a new prescription. (Remember to do this when you are getting low rather than waiting until you run out!)

What is a breath-actuated inhaler device?

Breath-actuated devices were developed to overcome the co-ordination problems of MDIs; they release the drug automatically as you breathe in through the mouthpiece, thus removing the

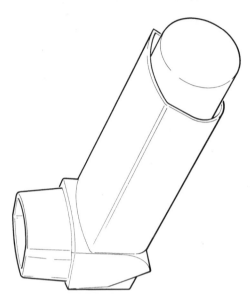

Figure 6.1 How to use a metered-dose inhaler (puffer).

1 Remove the cap and shake the inhaler.
2 Breathe out gently.
3 Put the mouthpiece in your mouth. At the start of inhaling (breathing in), which should be slow and deep, press the canister down
   and continue to inhale (breathe in) deeply.
4 Hold your breath for about 10 seconds, or for as long as
   possible.
5 Wait about 30 seconds before taking another inhalation.

need to press and breathe at the same time. There are two breath-
actuated devices available: the Autohaler (Figure 6.2) and the
Easi-Breathe (Figure 6.3).

Like MDIs, breath-actuated devices should be stored away
from extremes of temperature. Similarly, if the mouthpiece gets
dirty, clean it with a damp cloth. They, too, should be replaced
when empty. Remember to get a new prescription when the
device is getting low rather than when you've run out.

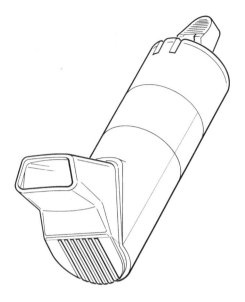

Figure 6.2 How to use the Autohaler.

1 Remove the protective mouthpiece and shake the inhaler.
2 Hold the inhaler upright and push the lever right up.
3 Breathe out gently. Keep the inhaler upright and put the mouthpiece in your mouth and close your lips round it. (Do not block the air holes with your hand.)
4 Breathe in steadily through your mouth. Don't stop breathing when the inhaler 'clicks' but continue taking a really deep breath.
5 Hold your breath for about 10 seconds.

NB The lever must be pushed up ('on') before each dose and pushed down ('off') again afterwards; otherwise it won't operate.

What is a dry powder inhaler?

This type of inhaler gives the drug in the form of a dry powder. It does not require co-ordination but still needs a good technique to be sure that as much as possible of the drug reaches the lungs – optimum drug delivery. Some devices such as the Aerohaler and

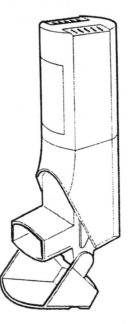

Figure 6.3 How to use the Easi-Breathe.

1 Shake the inhaler.
2 Hold the inhaler upright. Open the cap.
3 Breathe out gently. Keep the inhaler upright, put the mouthpiece in your mouth and close your lips and teeth round it (do not cover the air holes on the top with your hand).
4 Breathe in steadily through the mouthpiece. Don't stop breathing when the inhaler 'puffs' but continue taking a really deep breath.
5 Hold your breath for about 10 seconds.
6 After use, hold the inhaler upright and immediately close the cap.
7 For a second dose, wait a few seconds before repeating steps 1–6

HandiHaler are used with capsules that may be affected by the atmosphere if they are not stored correctly, away from extremes of temperature and protected from damp. The Diskhaler has a set dose of powdered medication fixed into a circular disk protected by a thin foil. The disk is inserted into the device itself. Because

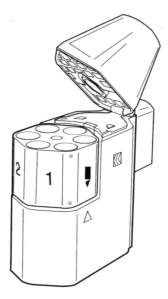

Figure 6.4 How to use the Aerohaler.

To load
1 Open the mouthpiece by lifting it up.
2 Lift the magazine up slightly and turn it round in a clockwise direction until the mark 6 lines up with the △ on the base. Push the magazine down again.
3 Load the capsules (either way up) into the magazine. Push the mouthpiece down until it clicks.

To use
1 Hold the inhaler upright. Push the white button on the side of the inhaler until it clicks and then release it immediately. (This pierces the capsule.)
2 Breathe out gently, put the mouthpiece in your mouth and breathe in as deeply as possible.
3 Remover the Aerohaler from your mouth and hold your breath for about 10 seconds. Then breathe out gently.
4 Turn the magazine until the next lowest number appears above the mark △ on the base. The next dose is now ready.
5 Reload the magazine when all the capsules have been used.

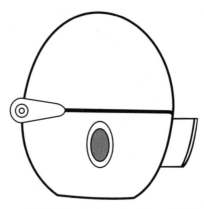

Figure 6.5 How to use the HandiHaler.

1 Remove the capsule from the blister pack it is supplied in. The capsules should always be stored in the sealed blisters and removed only immediately before use.
2 Open the dust cap of the HandiHaler by pulling it upwards, then open the mouthpiece.
3 Place the capsule in the centre chamber. (It does not matter which end of the capsule is placed in the chamber.)
4 Close the mouthpiece firmly until you hear a click, leaving the dust cap open.
5 Hold the HandiHaler with the mouthpiece upwards and press the piercing button completely in once and then release. This makes holes in the capsule and allows the medication to be released when you breathe in.
6 Breathe out completely. It is important to not breathe into the mouthpiece at any time.
7 Place the HandiHaler in your mouth and close your lips tightly around the mouthpiece. Keep your head upright and breathe in slowly and deeply, at a rate sufficient to hear the capsule vibrate, until your lungs are full. Hold your breath for as long as is comfortable and at the same time take the HandiHaler out of your mouth. Resume normal breathing.
8 After you have taken your dose, open the mouthpiece and tip out the used capsule and dispose of it.
9 Close the mouthpiece and dust cap to store the device.

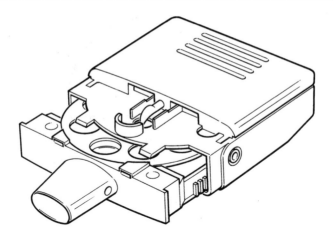

Figure 6.6 How to use the Diskhaler.

To load
1   Remove the mouthpiece cover, then remove the white tray by pulling it out gently and then squeezing the white ridges either side until it slides out.
2   Put the foil disk – numbers uppermost – on the wheel and slide the tray back.
3   Holding the corners of the tray, slide the tray in and out to rotate the disk until the highest number shows in the window.
To use
1   Keeping the device level, lift the rear of the lid up as far as it will go. This will pierce the top and bottom of the blister. Close the lid.
2   Holding the device level, breathe out gently and put the mouthpiece in your mouth. Breathe in as deeply as possible. (Do not cover the small air holes on either side of the mouthpiece.)
3   Remove the device from your mouth and hold your breath for about 10 seconds.
4   Slide the tray in and out ready for the next dose.

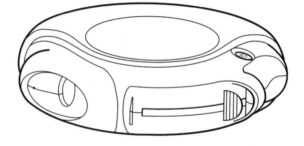

Figure 6.7 How to use the Accuhaler.

1 Hold the outer casing of the device in one hand while pushing the thumb grip away until you hear a click.
2 Holding the device with the mouthpiece towards you, slide the lever away until it clicks. This makes the dose available for inhalation and moves the dose counter on.
3 Keeping the device level, breathe out gently away from it, put the mouthpiece in your mouth and suck in steadily and deeply.
4 Remove the device from your mouth and hold your breath for about 10 seconds.
5 To close, slide the thumb grip back towards you as far as it will go, until it clicks.
6 For a second dose, repeat steps 1–5.

each dose is sealed in foil it is less likely to be affected by atmospheric conditions. The Accuhaler, Clickhaler and Turbohaler are multi-dose dry powder devices that contain the drug in the device.

Each dry powder device requires a slightly different inhaler technique and has different care and cleaning instructions. They are shown in Figures 6.4 through 6.9, with instructions on how to use them.

Some Turbohalers that contain a drug called Symbicort (budesonide) have been updated and now have a dose counter that counts backwards so you know how many doses are left.

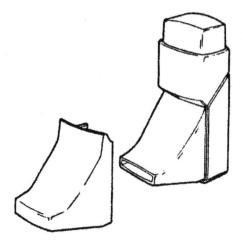

Figure 6.8 How to use the Clickhaler.

1 Hold the Clickhaler upright.
2 Remove the mouthpiece from the inhaler.
3 Shake the inhaler.
4 Continue to hold the Clickhaler upright with your thumb on the base and a finger on the coloured push-button.
5 Press the dosing button down firmly – once only – and then release.
6 Breathe out gently and put the mouthpiece between your lips and teeth, sealing your lips round the mouthpiece (do not breathe out into the Clickhaler).
7 Breathe in steadily and deeply. Remove the Clickhaler from your mouth and hold your breath for about 5–10 seconds. Breathe out slowly.
8 For a second dose, keep the Clickhaler upright and repeat steps 3–7.
9 Replace the mouthpiece cover after use.
10 There is a dose counter at the back of the inhaler. After 190 actuations, a red warning appears in the counter window, which shows that there are 10 actuations left. When no actuations are left, the inhaler locks; it can no longer be used and should be discarded.

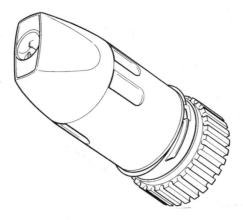

Figure 6.9 How to use the Turbohaler.

1 Unscrew and lift off the white cover. Hold the device upright and twist the grip forwards and backwards as far as it will go. You should hear a click.
2 Breathe out gently, put the mouthpiece between your lips and breathe in as deeply as possible. Even when you take a full dose, there may be no taste.
3 Remove the device from your mouth and hold your breath for about 10 seconds.
4 Replace the white cover.

Some Turbohalers that contain a drug called Symbicort (budesonide) have been updated and now have a dose counter that counts backwards so you know how many doses are left.

You mention that I could use a spacer device in my inhaler. What is that?

Spacer devices are add-on chambers that are used with MDIs. They increase the space between the inhaler and your mouth, and have three main advantages:

- They make MDIs easier to use effectively and can be as effective as a nebuliser.

- More drug gets into the lungs, where it is needed.
- There is less chance of side-effects. With ordinary inhalers, a lot of the drug ends up in the mouth where it is swallowed and absorbed into the bloodstream, which may lead to side-effects. Some drugs, such as inhaled steroids, can occasionally cause a hoarse voice or thrush in the mouth; using a spacer reduces this risk.

If you use a spacer, it is vital that you inhale from the device as soon as possible after actuating the MDI, because the drug is in aerosol form for only a very short time. You should take one puff at a time; leave a gap of 30–60 seconds between puffs if you are prescribed more. Shake the MDI between each puff.

To use the spacer, attach it to your MDI, place the mouthpiece of the spacer into your mouth, sealing your lips round the mouthpiece, and then press the canister to release one puff of your medication. You may be advised to follow one or other of two methods for breathing in the drug through the spacer:

- after pressing the canister, take one deep breath in and hold it for 5–10 seconds;
- alternatively, after pressing the canister, breathe in and out slowly and gently four or five times for each puff (this is known as *tidal breathing*).

Each method is as effective as the other. Your doctor or nurse will advise you which technique is better for you.

Spacer devices should be cleaned once a month by washing in mild detergent, rinsing and allowing to air dry. Never wipe them dry as this increases the electrostatic charge (static), which may make the aerosol drug stick to the sides of the spacer and lessen the effectiveness of your treatment.

The Able Spacer, the AeroChamber, the Nebuhaler and the Volumatic are shown in Figures 6.10 through 6.13, with instructions on how to use them.

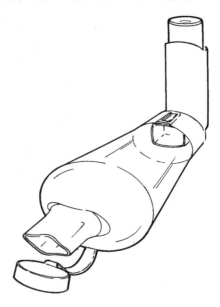

Figure 6.10 How to use the Able spacer.

1   Remove the mouthpiece cap from both the Able spacer and the metered-dose inhaler (MDI).
2   Place the MDI into the end of the Able spacer that does not have the cap attached.
3   Make sure that you push it in fully.
4   Shake the spacer and MDI together two or three times.
5   Place the mouthpiece in your mouth, closing your lips tightly round the mouthpiece.
6   Breathe out normally and then press down firmly on the canister, releasing one dose of medication. Breathe in slowly and deeply. If the 'coaching' device on the spacer sounds, you are breathing in too fast.
7   Remove the spacer from your mouth while continuing to hold your breath for 5–10 seconds. Then breathe out normally.
8   After use, remove the MDI from the spacer and replace the cap on the MDI as well as the cap on the spacer. The MDI can be stored inside the Able spacer.
9   If you need another dose of medicine, repeat steps 4–7.

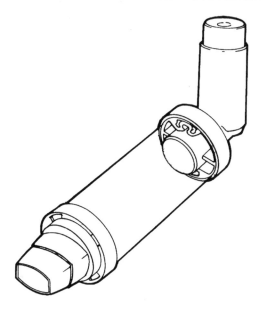

Figure 6.11 How to use the AeroChamber.

1 Remove the cap.
2 Shake the inhaler and insert it into the back of the AeroChamber
3 Place the mouthpiece in your mouth (or the mask over your mouth and nose).
4 Press the canister once to release a dose of the drug.
5 Take a deep, slow breath in. (If you hear a whistling sound, you are breathing in too quickly.)
6 Hold your breath for about 10 seconds; then breathe out through the mouthpiece.
7 Breathe in again but do not press the canister.
8 Remove the mouthpiece from your mouth and breathe out.
9 Wait a few seconds before you take a second dose, and repeat steps 2–8.

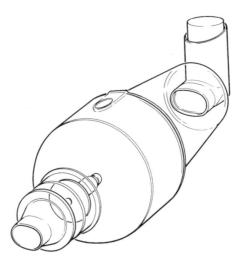

Figure 6.12 How to use the Nebuhaler spacer device.

1 Remove the cap, shake the inhaler and insert it into the device.
2 Place the mouthpiece in your mouth (make sure that your lips are *behind* the ring).
3 Breathe in and out slowly and gently (there will be a clicking sound as the valve opens and closes).
4 Once your breathing pattern is well established, depress the canister and leave the device in the same position while you continue to breathe (called tidal breathing) several more times.
5 Remove the device from your mouth.
6 Wash the device and leave it to dry – never wipe it dry.

A friend who also has COPD is on a different kind of inhaler. Why is this?

The most likely reason is that your doctor or nurse has selected the most suitable inhaler device for you. There are many different devices that offer the same type of drug, but do so in different ways. The metered-dose inhaler (MDI) is still the most commonly prescribed but many people have difficulty with it because they

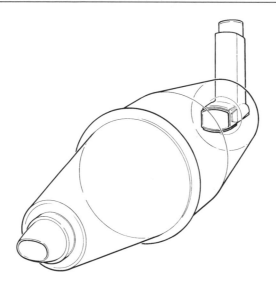

Figure 6.13 How to use the Volumatic spacer device.

1 Remove the cap.
2 Shake the inhaler and insert it into the device.
3 Place the mouthpiece in your mouth.
4 Start breathing in and out slowly and gently. (This will make a clicking sound as the valve opens and closes.)
5 Once your breathing pattern is well established, depress the canister, leaving the device in the same position and continue to breathe (tidal breathing) several more times.
6 Remove the device from your mouth.
7 Wait about 30 seconds before repeating steps 2–6.
8 Wash the device and leave it to dry – never wipe it dry.

can't co-ordinate their breathing with the release of the spray. The breath-actuated and dry powder devices do not require such good co-ordination, and so are easier to use correctly.

Your doctor or nurse should help you to find the type of device that suits you best. After all, you are the person who has to take the treatment, and you need to be happy with the device. What suits one person will not necessarily suit another, so there is no reason why your friend who also has COPD should not be on an inhaler device different from yours.

Can I get another device from my doctor if I am not happy with my present inhaler?

This should not be a problem. There is a wide range of inhaler devices available for COPD treatment, so it is not necessary to continue with one you do not get on with. The best approach would be to make an appointment with your practice nurse. Most surgeries keep a selection of inhaler devices, so you can see what is available and try them out. As long as the same type of drug is available, you should be able to switch. Once you have agreed on which device suits you, and that you can use it correctly, you can change to that for your regular prescription.

Where can I go to get someone to show me how to use my inhaler properly?

You can get help with this problem from a number of places. A chest or asthma clinic at your GP's practice would be ideal. Although not all practices run such clinics, your GP or practice nurse should be able to help. If you are a hospital patient, the specialist respiratory nurse or physiotherapist will be able to help you. Your pharmacist may also be able to supply you with a leaflet and some practical help.

Walk-in centres are being set up all over the country as part of the Government policy of modernisation for the NHS. The nurses who staff these 'one-stop shops' should be able to help you. NHS Direct can give advice by telephone, but seeing the inhaler demonstrated one-to-one is probably better. Finally, Breathe Easy, the patient arm of the British Lung Foundation, has groups all over the UK with members who are very experienced in the practicalities of coping with COPD.

How will I know when my MDI is running low?

It is not always easy to tell how much remains in the canister but shaking the MDI gently can give you an idea as to how full it is. Over time you will get a feel for how much is left. If you still are unsure whether your MDI is running low, ask your pharmacist to check to see if you need to order a new one.

Occasionally, the hole through which the drug is delivered can become blocked with deposits of drug particles. A common reason for this can be condensation, especially if you tend to breathe in and out of the inhaler mouthpiece several times before you press the canister. It is important to clean the inhaler regularly, as described in the manufacturer's 'patient information leaflet' supplied with the inhaler. Never attempt to unblock the hole with a pin, as this can alter the size of the aerosol spray and make your treatment less effective.

Nebulisers

A nebuliser may be the best way to deliver medication to your lungs if you cannot use any of the inhaler devices or spacers described above to relieve or treat your COPD, or if your symptoms have become severe and are not relieved using regular doses of medication. The fine mist a nebuliser creates safely allows smaller particles of medication to be breathed in efficiently and in a higher dose when your symptoms cannot be controlled with inhaler devices. Although most people with COPD use nebulised medication to control symptoms and give quick relief of breathlessness, a minority may also be prescribed 'preventer' treatment including steroid therapy, or antibiotics to control persistent infection in the airways.

Nebulisers should be used only if recommended by a doctor. Anyone with COPD who is thought to need one will be thoroughly assessed; if the person benefits from a trial with nebulisers, a nebuliser system will often be recommended. You should not buy a nebuliser without discussing it first with your doctor, as it might not be suitable or appropriate for you. Nebuliser systems are not usually available on the NHS and cost from about £120. Some hospitals now offer a nebuliser loan service; however, the provision of this service is patchy and you need to be referred to the service for an assessment before a nebuliser will be provided.

My doctor is sending me for an assessment for a nebuliser. What will be involved?

A nebuliser assessment is usually carried out to see if you get more benefit from your medication when it is given by a nebuliser than you do with your inhalers. You will be asked to try different combinations of drugs over a number of weeks, at home. A typical trial runs for four to eight weeks and usually consists of:

- Weeks 1 and 2: high doses of bronchodilators in combination through a spacer; e.g. salbutamol 4 puffs four times a day, with ipratropium bromide 4 puffs four times a day.
- Weeks 3 and 4: salbutamol four times a day through the nebuliser.
- Weeks 5 and 6: ipratropium bromide four times a day through the nebuliser.
- Weeks 7 and 8: salbutamol and ipratropium bromide four times a day through the nebuliser.

You are usually asked to keep a record of your peak flow and symptoms, effects and side-effects during the trial. At the end of the assessment period you and your doctor will be able to judge whether you will benefit from a nebuliser and, if so, which drugs should be used. You will then be supplied with all the necessary equipment to use the device at home.

Despite everyone's best efforts to try to find out who would benefit from a nebuliser, the research in this area is pretty scanty and there are some hospitals that don't think nebulisers should be used at home at all! In other areas people are given nebulisers if they are coming into hospital (e.g. four admissions over a 12-month period). The position is likely to change over the next few years, so what we tell you today may not be what happens tomorrow.

What actually is a nebuliser?

A nebuliser system is a machine driven by an electrically powered compressor that drives air into a chamber holding a liquid form of medication. The air breaks up the liquid into tiny droplets, forming a mist that you can then breathe into your lungs. Although many people with lung problems such as COPD and asthma feel that a nebuliser is a magical device, it is important to realise that it is no more than a very effective way of delivering standard treatment. You should also be aware that a nebuliser can be tricky to put together. It needs cleaning and servicing regularly and lacks the portability of inhaler devices; spacer devices are highly effective in delivering drugs into the lungs and are easier to use and look after than a nebuliser. However, nebulised therapy can be a more effective treatment for some people with severe COPD.

There are two main sorts of nebuliser systems in current use, the jet nebuliser and the ultrasonic nebuliser.

Jet nebuliser systems (Figure 6.14) are electrically powered and are available in portable versions. They work by forcing a stream of compressed air through a fine nozzle into a nebulising chamber. The drug solution is drawn up into the chamber and broken into particles of mist. You inhale the tiny particles, while the larger droplets fall back into the bottom of the chamber and are then re-nebulised.

Ultrasonic nebuliser systems also produce an aerosol mist but by a different method. Ultrasound waves break up the drug solution into a fine spray. These nebulisers are very quiet, portable and deliver the drug quickly, but can be expensive, costing up to £200. They are not usually available from hospital nebuliser clinics and, although very easy to use, are not suitable in all situations.

There are other types of specialised nebuliser systems but you should not go out and buy or hire a nebuliser without first discussing it carefully with your doctor.

What is the difference between a nebuliser and a compressor?

We often mistakenly refer to a compressor as a nebuliser, which makes things confusing. In fact, the small pot that you put your

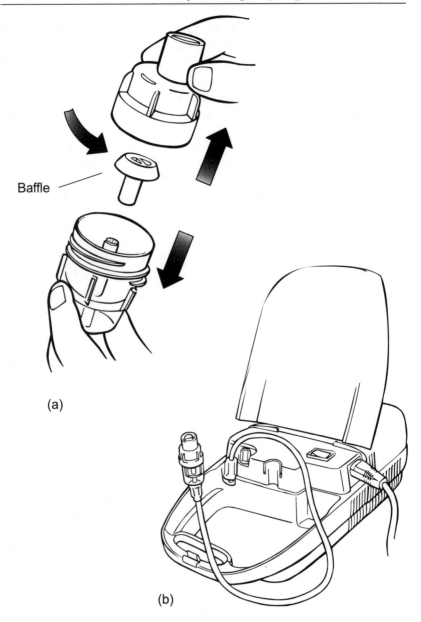

Baffle

(a)

(b)

Figure 6.14 Examples of (a) a nebuliser and (b) a compressor.

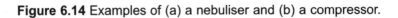

medication into is actually the nebuliser and the compressor is the electrically powered machine that provides pressurised air to it. This nebulising chamber is where the liquid drug is turned into a fine mist or aerosol that you can inhale into your lungs. The system will not work without the baffle (see Figure 6.14a), which is a vital part of the nebulising chamber. You must take care not to lose or misplace it.

The drugs used in your nebuliser chamber are available on prescription through the NHS. However, often the compressor and nebuliser chambers are not. Nebulisers start at around £120 and chambers cost between £2.50 and £5.00 each, depending on their make and durability.

How do I use my nebuliser and compressor system properly?

Whether you have been advised to purchase, hire or borrow a compressor with a nebuliser unit, make sure you understand all the practical details: how to use it, how to keep it clean and how to maintain it. You should be given written instructions that cover all these aspects so that you can refer to it when needed. Perhaps the best way of ensuring that you understand exactly how to use the unit correctly is to practise putting the whole system together with your doctor or nurse. Having a member of your family present at the practice session might be sensible, as they can help you to remember all the details.

When you use a compressor put it on a clean hard surface, such as a table. Keeping the compressor off the floor will help stop dust getting inside. To take your medication you should sit comfortably in an upright position and breathe gently. Do not try to breathe too quickly or too deeply: the treatment should not be hard work. If you need a break half way through, you can switch off the compressor. Most nebulisers usually take 5–10 minutes from switching on to deliver the drug. The nebulisation period is over when the liquid in the chamber starts to spit. Tap the chamber to shake down any large droplets and continue to nebulise for a further minute. At the end of this time there will be a small amount of liquid left in the chamber; this is normal. If your nebuliser takes much longer to deliver the mist, there could be a problem and you should ask your nebuliser supplier for advice.

How do I look after my nebuliser and compressor?

It is essential to keep your nebuliser and compressor system clean and in good working order.

* Keep the compressor on a clean firm surface such as a table, because dusty air will be drawn into the machine if it is kept on the carpet or floor.
* Do not block the ventilation holes.
* Keep the compressor clean by wiping it with a damp cloth.

In general, have your compressor checked and serviced at least once a year. The nebulising chamber may need to be changed every two months unless you have a durable chamber (usually grey coloured), which will last for a year. Find out how to change the inlet filter (and outlet filter, if one is fitted). You can find out about this from the manufacturer, a pharmacist or your local lung function laboratory at the hospital. Filters should be changed every three months, but more often if they become discoloured. Nebuliser tubing, masks and mouthpieces should also be changed every three months unless, again, they are durable, in which case they will last for a year. If you are unsure how long your chamber, tubing, mask or mouthpiece will last, ask your doctor or nurse for advice.

You will also need to ask about service arrangements and emergency provision if your compressor develops a fault. Some hospitals have a nebuliser service that provides help and advice about the care of nebulisers; contact your local hospital to see if they offer this. In case your compressor fails, you should have a back-up such as an inhaler with a spacer device; ask your doctor about this.

While your compressor is being serviced you will be without one. You may find that the manufacturer will lend you one. Alternatively, check with your doctor or nurse to see if they will lend you one during this time. Some pharmacies have a nebuliser service that includes the hire of compressors.

How do I clean my nebuliser chamber?

It is important to keep your nebuliser clean and dry, as germs may grow in damp equipment. A small amount of drug always remains in the chamber after treatment. This can block the nebuliser jets if it is not cleaned. To keep your system working safely and effectively, follow these steps.

- After every use disconnect the nebuliser from the tubing and turn on the compressor for a short period to clear any moisture from the tubing.
- Remove the mouthpiece or mask from the nebuliser. Unscrew the nebuliser. Take care not to lose the baffle (see Figure 6.14a), as the nebuliser will not work without it.
- Wash the nebuliser and mouthpiece/mask in hot soapy water (washing-up liquid is fine). Rinse them under hot running water to clear the fine jet holes and dry thoroughly with a clean cloth or leave in a dry place.
- It is essential that the nebuliser parts are completely dry before they are reassembled.
- Change the nebuliser chamber, tubing and mouthpiece/ mask every three months, unless they are of the more durable type (see next point).
- For nebuliser chambers that are more durable and will last for 12 months, follow the cleaning instructions above. Then, to sterilise them and ensure maximum performance, they should be boiled with two drops of washing up liquid for 5–10 minutes after every 30 uses (about once a week). If you are uncertain whether your nebuliser is durable, ask your doctor, nurse or the manufacturer.

Can I use my nebuliser when I am travelling?

Most nebuliser and compressor systems can be used away from home. You can plug your system into a mains supply when you travel anywhere in the UK. If you are going abroad, find out whether the mains supply is compatible or if you will need an adapter. There are a number of systems that operate from a 12-volt DC car cigarette lighter socket or from a battery. You may be able to hire these from manufacturers, hospitals and some pharmacies.

Check that your insurance will cover your equipment, and any complications you may have while away. If you are travelling abroad, ask your doctor for a letter outlining your need for medication in case you are stopped at Customs. Make sure that you have enough medicine and accessories to cover you for the time that you are away, plus a little longer in case you are delayed on your return.

You can travel with your nebuliser and compressor system on an aeroplane. Some airlines will allow you to use a battery-operated system and some carry their own. Check with the airline before you book and make sure you inform them of all your requirements.

7
Oxygen therapy

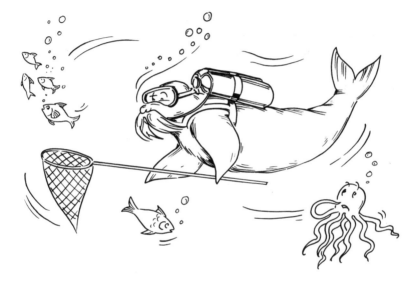

If sufficient damage is done to the airways and the air sacs, not enough oxygen gets into the bloodstream. This 'low blood oxygen' is called *hypoxaemia* and is associated with impaired function of nearly all the other organs in the body, but particularly the heart. A more common medical term is *hypoxia*, which also implies too little oxygen. We will use this term from now on. Hypoxia can occur as a consequence of severe COPD or during a flare-up of the condition. This chapter covers the use of oxygen in both situations.

Oxygen in the acute attack

During a flare-up of COPD the airways are more inflamed and so less oxygen is delivered to the lungs' air sacs (alveoli) for gas exchange. If the flare-up is associated with pneumonia, there may also be damage to the air sacs themselves. Depending on the severity of the attack, this damage may be sufficient to cause hypoxia.

My partner's GP mentioned something about respiratory failure. What is this?

'Respiratory failure' is a broad term which really means that the process of breathing is not working efficiently. It has a variety of causes, ranging from problems with the breathing muscles themselves (muscular dystrophy, for example), right the way through to damage to the lungs themselves (as in severe emphysema). In medical terms, we divide respiratory failure into type I and type II, on the basis of calculations of the levels of oxygen and carbon dioxide in the person's blood (the 'blood oxygen and carbon dioxide levels').

- In *type I* failure the blood oxygen level is low but the blood carbon dioxide level is normal.
- In *type II* failure not only is the blood oxygen level low but the blood carbon dioxide level is raised as well. (Carbon dioxide is the 'waste gas' that we breathe out; in severe cases of respiratory failure the amount of carbon dioxide can build up in your blood.)

What are the signs of low blood oxygen?

An increase in your breathing sufficient to make it difficult for you to speak implies a severe attack of low blood oxygen. A purple or blue discolouration around your tongue and mouth or of your fingernails can also be associated with low blood oxygen. When the blood oxygen level falls, people can become confused or disorientated.

If any of the above occurs, seek medical attention immediately.

If it's important to know how much oxygen is in the blood, how is it measured?

A measurement of the percentage of oxygen saturating your blood can now be measured by finger probe (like a plastic clothes-peg placed on the end of your finger). This value is called *oxygen saturation*. It can be measured in some GP surgeries, by ambulance staff and in all hospitals. To get a more accurate measurement of blood oxygen a sample of blood has to be taken, either from one of your arteries or from the capillary vessels of an earlobe.

I find it hard to get to my local hospital. Can't I do this oxygen measurement at home the way people with diabetes check their blood sugar?

It is possible to buy equipment to measure oxygen saturation, but it is very expensive and will probably make you worry more than it will help in the management of your COPD. If your doctor or nurse thinks it important to monitor your oxygen saturation at home, it is possible for your local hospital to arrange this. However, you will need to be reviewed by a chest specialist first, as the vast majority of people do not need to have these measurements done regularly.

Blood gas measurements are almost always done in hospital because the sample needs to be analysed immediately.

My dad was in hospital when he had a bad turn, and I heard the nurse talk about possibly giving him NIPPV. What is it?

This stands for **N**asal **I**ntermittent **P**ositive-**P**ressure **V**entilation. It is a special treatment used in hospital for people who have sufficiently severe attacks of COPD that they cannot breathe well enough on their own. This treatment is used only with very ill people, probably less than 5 per cent of those admitted to hospital with exacerbations of COPD.

Basically, what happens is this. A special mask is attached to your face, which completely covers your nose and sometimes your mouth as well. It is connected to a machine that can sense you breathing in and out. At the start of your breath in, the machine drives the oxygen down into your lungs more efficiently than you would otherwise be able to do on your own, and helps you to breathe out more efficiently, too.

Normally, people who have NIPPV need it only at the beginning of their time in hospital. It may sound a bit claustrophobic but it's only a treatment used in particularly difficult situations, and at these times people are usually glad to receive it.

Do I need to have oxygen at home to help me through an acute attack?

Oxygen at home is usually considered only for people with severe COPD (see the 'Spirometry' section in Chapter 3, *How is COPD diagnosed?*). If you have a severe attack of COPD, there are a number of treatments in addition to oxygen that should help you through it, so our advice would be to seek immediate medical attention. Any attack severe enough for you to need oxygen might require you to attend hospital.

If you have an attack sufficiently severe to require admission to hospital, it is likely that the medical team looking after you will measure your oxygen levels. This is often done on the day of your admission and again when you are a lot better. Decisions about oxygen use at home are usually made sometime after the 'acute' stage, usually at a hospital clinic visit.

My friend was recently brought home from hospital by a special nurse. She said that she was part of an 'ARAS' team. What is this?

'ARAS' stands for **A**cute **R**espiratory **A**ssessment **S**ervice, and is a relatively new innovation in the management of COPD. It is a service provided by hospitals to enable them to look after people with sudden deteriorations of their COPD, at home. Normally these people would have to be admitted to hospital for monitoring but ARAS team members are able to regularly review people in their own home and monitor the effectiveness of treatment in a similar way to that done by nurses in hospitals. Because the team members are particularly experienced in respiratory medicine and COPD in particular, the level of care is often more specialised than that received in hospital.

ARAS team members are able to offer nebulisers and oxygen for people at home to help them through deteriorations in COPD. If someone fails to respond to treatment, though, they can then be admitted to hospital.

If you are seen by the ARAS service, you are typically visited for up to ten days. At the end of this period, a decision is taken as to whether you will be followed up by the hospital or your GP, or both.

Oxygen for long-term use

My wife's doctor said that there's a possibility that she'll be given an oxygen concentrator. What is it, and what does it do?

An oxygen concentrator is a machine about the size of a small shopping trolley (see Figure 7.1), which is fitted into your house and allows your wife to have oxygen available whenever she needs it, for as long as she wants. The machine takes in room air and filters out all the other gases except oxygen, allowing pure oxygen to come out of the other end – it literally 'concentrates' oxygen from room air. Tubing is attached to allow oxygen to be available anywhere in your home. It's a bit like plumbing-in a boiler for central heating and then running pipes from it to make sure every room is kept warm. But instead of having radiators you have 'oxygen points' into which you can attach tubing for oxygen, similar to that used if your wife needs oxygen when she is admitted to hospital.

I've heard of a machine called an oxygen concentrator, which sounds as though it would be really helpful for me. How can I get one?

There is a particular group of people with COPD who are helped considerably by receiving oxygen therapy regularly. They are people with severe disease and those in whom damage to the

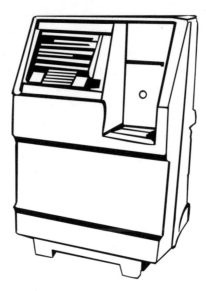

Figure 7.1 An oxygen concentrator.

lungs is beginning to affect their heart. Severe COPD means that your lungs do not allow sufficient oxygen to get into your bloodstream. As well as making you feel breathless, this low level of oxygen affects the performance of your heart, particularly by increasing the pressure on the right side of the heart. You may notice swelling of your ankles if this happens.

The medical term for severe COPD causing low oxygen and changes to the performance of your heart is *cor pulmonale*. Cor pulmonale occurs late on in COPD and is a particularly important feature as it signals the need for people to receive daily therapy with oxygen.

Unlike with 'acute' attacks of COPD, where oxygen is used to get you through the short-term problem, someone with cor pulmonale needs oxygen therapy every day for a minimum of 16 hours out of every 24. This may seem like an awful lot but a number of studies have found that this is the minimum length of time that your heart needs to receive this extra oxygen to help it beat properly. Also, it is a treatment you will need every day, regardless of whether you feel 'stable' or not.

I understand that an oxygen concentrator is not always appropriate but how will I know whether I will need one?

It is only people with low oxygen levels every day who require oxygen every day from a concentrator, so you need not worry unless you have severe disease (FEV_1 less than 30% predicted – see the 'Spirometry' section in Chapter 3). The most recent guidelines issued to doctors recommend that people with severe COPD should have their oxygen levels measured. Many people with severe COPD have suffered deterioration sufficient to require their attendance at the A&E department or even to be admitted to hospital. It is usually at this time that an assessment of oxygen level is made; if necessary, a more formal assessment of oxygen requirements can be made later on, when you are feeling more settled or more stable.

It is important that you are assessed for the need for an oxygen concentrator when you are relatively stable, because your oxygen measurements can be unusually low if you are in the middle of an infection. It is usual to take two measurements of oxygen, about three weeks apart.

My doctor has told me that I need an oxygen concentrator but I don't understand how the process will work. Can you advise me?

The process for getting an oxygen concentrator changed early in 2006; it is arranged by a specialist team after they have assessed you and decided that you need it. The assessment, which is almost always done at the hospital, involves checking your blood gases (oxygen levels) on and off oxygen to work out the correct amount of oxygen for you to use regularly at home. Very rarely, it may involve an overnight stay in hospital. The measurements should be done when you are relatively stable, because your oxygen levels can be unusually low if you are in the middle of an infection; they are usually done twice, with a gap of three weeks between measurements. In a few areas of the country it is possible to carry out this assessment in your home.

The specialist team then completes a Home Oxygen Order Form (known as a 'HOOF'!), which is similar to a doctor's prescription.

The HOOF contains all the information about your needs for oxygen, including the flow rate that the concentrator should be set at (usually 2, 3 or 4 litres per minute) and the minimum number of hours per day you are required to use the concentrator – normally 16 hours per day. The HOOF is then passed (with your consent) to a home oxygen supply company who will deliver and install your oxygen concentrator. A representative of the company will discuss with you the most suitable place to site the concentrator and any oxygen points. They will show you how everything works and answer any questions you have about the machine. They will also leave you a back-up cylinder of oxygen and a 24-hour contact number so that if you have any problems you can get them sorted straight away. They will return at regular intervals to service the machine and check it is working properly.

Someone from the specialist team will also contact you at regular intervals to check on your progress and offer you ongoing information and support. If you are having any problems you can contact them or speak to your GP or practice nurse.

I have been told to use my oxygen concentrator for 16 hours each day, but I can't work out the best times to use it.

The short answer is that you can use the concentrator whenever you like, provided that you use it for a minimum of 16 hours per day (that is, 16 hours out of *every* 24). Remember that this is a minimum recommendation; if you feel happier being on oxygen for longer than 16 hours, this is fine. However, most people worry about how to get 16 hours a day done! Here is a possible way to break it down.

- First make sure you use it at night. If you spend 8 hours in bed, you have used up half the time needed straight away.
- Another 3–5 hours can be spent in the evening – for example, while you are watching television.
- The remaining 3–5 hours can be 'cobbled together' through-out the morning and afternoon.

In this way you do not have to feel 'tied' to the house.

My doctor is reluctant to prescribe a concentrator for me, as I have not yet given up smoking. Is this really right?

Well, your doctor is correct about the fact that you should give up smoking, particularly as your disease is sufficiently severe to contemplate providing you with a concentrator. The main concern about people who smoke using a concentrator is the potential for them to receive nasty burns to their face and even start a fire. The current recommendations do not forbid your doctor to prescribe a concentrator for you but they do point out that every attempt should be made to stop you smoking before one is installed.

If you really cannot give up smoking, it is vital that you **always** remove the oxygen tubing or mask before you have a cigarette. We have seen the injuries inflicted by a combination of oxygen and a cigarette, and they are very painful!

I need oxygen to get around the house but I also want to get out. Is there any way I can take oxygen with me?

Yes, it is possible for you to have a small oxygen cylinder to use when you go out. As from 2006, people undergoing assessment for long-term oxygen therapy (LTOT) will also have their need for oxygen outside the home checked and, if required, this will be added to your HOOF and will be provided by the home oxygen supply company.

Portable cylinders vary in size and weight: broadly speaking, the larger the cylinder, the longer the oxygen lasts. In some cases a conserving device can be fitted to cylinders to extend their life but not everyone will benefit from this – some people cannot get enough oxygen using these devices. Your suitability for conserving devices will be checked at your assessment. If you are normally transported in a wheelchair it is usually possible to attach an oxygen cylinder to it.

I've heard of oxygen concentrators but what is liquid oxygen?

Liquid oxygen is another means by which oxygen can be provided in cylinders (as opposed to the usual gaseous form of oxygen). The advantage of liquid oxygen lies in the fact each cylinder lasts longer than oxygen in gaseous form. It is hoped that liquid oxygen will soon become available on the NHS. Until this happens, though, the best way of trying to get hold of liquid oxygen is to ask your doctor to contact the local primary care trust or health authority.

There is, however, no difference in the quality of the oxygen delivered. If you need oxygen at home, the gaseous form will be as good at giving you oxygen as the liquid form. The difference lies only in how long each cylinder lasts before it's empty. So why isn't everyone getting liquid oxygen? The simple answer is that it is much more expensive than conventional oxygen and so it's reserved for people who need oxygen for most of the day and also need to be out of their house for most of the day. If that person is you, talk to your doctor!

My dad uses an oxygen concentrator with nasal tubes instead of a mask. Why is this?

Nasal oxygen tubes – sometimes known as nasal prongs or cannulae (Figure 7.2) – are the best way to deliver long-term oxygen (more than 16 hours a day). They are less obtrusive than a mask, and also allow your dad to eat, drink or talk without removing them, which he would have to do if he were using a mask.

On the whole, they are comfortable to wear and easy to use. The ends of the prongs should be inserted gently into the nostrils for about 1–2 cm, with the tubing hooked over the ears and secured under the chin at the front. Occasionally, with long-term use, a few sore spots can appear, usually above the ears or on the cheeks. This can be avoided by padding the tubing in these areas with foam and preventing friction from the tube by securing it with sticking plaster. Specially designed foam pads and plasters are available for this purpose; your dad can ask his nurse or oxygen supply company for more details.

Some people develop soreness and dryness in the nostrils. This can be prevented by always inserting gently into the nostrils, not having the prongs too long, lubricating with non-flammable gel such as K-Y gel – but *not* Vaseline because it is flammable petro-

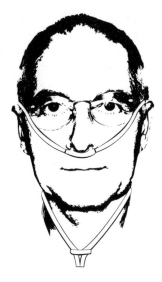

Figure 7.2 Nasal cannulae.

leum jelly) – and drinking plenty of fluids to avoid dehydration. If
your dad's nose becomes very sore, it may be appropriate for him
to switch to a mask until his nose heals and then revert to nasal
prongs, following all the advice above.

Will running an oxygen concentrator make my electricity bill higher?

No, it won't. There is a special meter inside the concentrator that
measures the running time. The electricity costs for running the
machine are refunded to you, so it costs you nothing!

8
Exercise and fitness

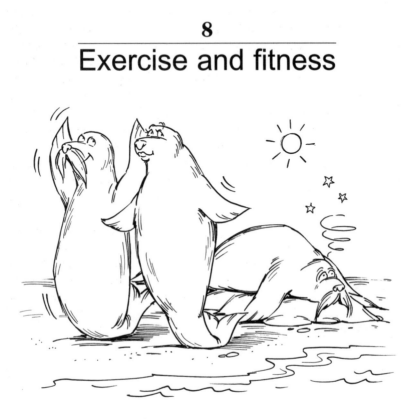

Physical exercise is an essential part of everyday life and is not harmful to people with COPD. It will improve your general fitness and give you a feeling of well-being. One of the main symptoms of COPD is breathlessness but, although this breathlessness may cause anxiety, it is *not* dangerous. Increasing your activity level and improving your fitness will, in a short period of time, reduce your sensation of breathlessness, not make it worse.

When you are at rest you normally take about 12–15 breaths a minute, giving you around 10–12 litres of air to supply your body with the oxygen it needs. When you move around and carry out any daily activity such as walking, cleaning or shopping, your lungs have to respond to your body's increasing requirement for oxygen. For you to be active, your muscles need to produce more energy, and to do this they need oxygen. Without oxygen your muscles easily become tired, making it harder to be active. People with COPD slowly begin to find that they cannot provide enough oxygen for their muscles to perform certain activities without feeling breathless. This breathlessness creeps up insidiously. Unless you do a lot of exercise or have a physically demanding job, you would not notice that you had a problem. This is the main reason why many people with COPD are not diagnosed until their condition has reached a more moderate or severe category.

Feeling breathless is unpleasant and can make you anxious. If you have noticed that you get breathless, you might have begun to adapt your lifestyle to prevent it: taking the car to the shops instead of walking and getting your partner to make the bed. But by reducing your level of activity, your muscles become de-conditioned and you will find it ever-more difficult to be active. When COPD becomes severe, even small amounts of activity such as walking slowly become difficult. This becomes a vicious downward cycle, but training your lungs and muscles can break it. By gradually building up the amount of exercise you do, you can help to improve your breathing and feel better.

Exercises to help breathing

I realise now that I must improve my fitness. How can I start?

Be sensible and build up gradually to prevent unnecessary breath-lessness. Start by walking a short distance and gradually increase the distance you walk, or the length of time you exercise. One of our patients used to count the number of lampposts he could get past before he needed a rest. Within a few weeks of daily walks he could get from his home to the surgery without a stop!

Even if your COPD is more severe, it is worth keeping as active as possible. Begin slowly by doing gentle arm and leg movements while you are sitting down. Then set a target such as walking from one room to another, to the front door, into the garden.

Try not to let your COPD stop you doing things. Try to keep up with household chores and gentle gardening for exercise. In particular, don't give up your social life or going on holiday; they are good for you and giving them up could put an extra burden on your partner or family. Do all of this and you will be surprised at how quickly you can improve. The more you manage, the less breathlessness and fear of becoming breathless you will experience and the better will be your quality of life.

Are there any exercises I can do at home to help my breathing?

Yes, there are. There is no need to go to a gym to improve your muscle strength and general fitness. A combination of strengthening exercise and 'aerobic' activity such as walking will give you the best kind of exercise programme. Try to get as much exercise as you can manage comfortably. Don't be afraid of getting out of breath: the more you can get your lungs working the better – but don't overdo it. Below are a series of reconditioning exercises that you can try at home. Do them regularly; it is surprising how quickly you will be able to do more!

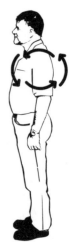

1 Shoulder shrugging
Circle your shoulders forward, down, backward and up. Try to keep your timing regular, allowing two full seconds per circle and relax throughout. Continue for 30 seconds. Repeat three times, with a short rest in between.

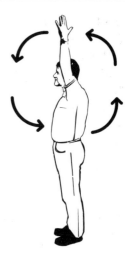

2 Full arm circling

One arm at a time, pass your arm as near as possible to the side of your head; move your arm in as large a circle as possible. Take about 10 seconds per circle and try to keep going for about 40 seconds. Repeat the exercise three times, with a short rest in between.

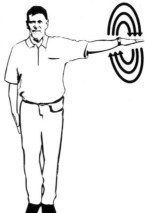

3 Increasing arm circles

Hold one arm away from your body at shoulder height and move it in a small circle. Progressively increase the size of the circle for a count of six circles in 10 seconds, and then decrease for a further count of six. Repeat for 40 seconds. Now do the same with the other arm.

4 Abdominal exercise

Sit upright but comfortably in a chair. Tighten your abdominal muscles by pulling your tummy button in and up towards your back. Hold for a count of four and then release over a count of four. Repeat continuously for 30 seconds. Do this exercise three times, with a short rest in between.

5 Wall press-ups

Stand with your feet a full arm's length away from the wall. Now place your hands on the wall and slowly bend your elbows until your nose touches the wall. Push your arms straight again, allowing about 8 seconds from start to completion. Repeat continuously for 40 seconds to a total of five repetitions. Repeat the exercise three times, with a short rest in between.

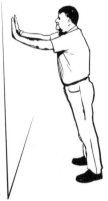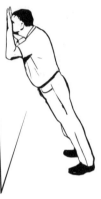

6 Sitting to standing

Using a dining chair, sit, stand and sit, allowing 10 seconds from start to completion. Repeat continuously for 40 seconds to a total of five repetitions. Do the exercise three times, with a short rest in between.

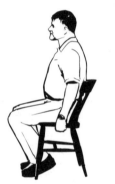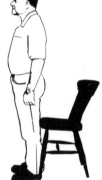

7 Quadriceps exercise

Sitting on a chair, straighten your right knee and tense your thigh muscles; hold for a count of four and then relax/lower your foot to the ground over a count of four. Try to do a total of five repetitions over 40 seconds. Repeat the exercise three times, with a short rest in between. Now repeat the exercise with your left leg.

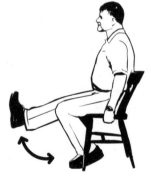

8 Calf exercise
Stand upright, holding
onto the back of a chair,
and rise up on your
toes and then back
down to the floor,
taking 8–10
seconds.
Repeat this
continuously for
40 seconds.

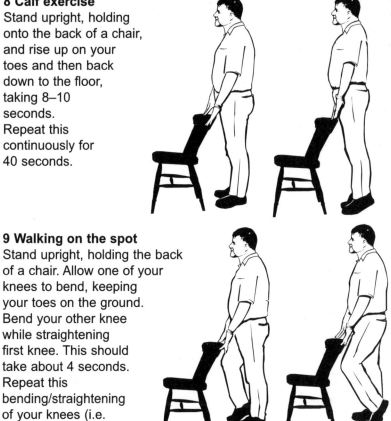

9 Walking on the spot
Stand upright, holding the back
of a chair. Allow one of your
knees to bend, keeping
your toes on the ground.
Bend your other knee
while straightening
first knee. This should
take about 4 seconds.
Repeat this
bending/straightening
of your knees (i.e.
walking on the spot),
always keeping your toes on the ground, for 40 seconds – ten times.
Repeat the exercise three times, with a short rest in between.

10 Step-ups
This can be done on a low step or the bottom stair. Over about 4
seconds step up with one foot onto the step and then bring up the
other foot, step down with the first foot and then the other foot; keep
going continuously for 40 seconds. Repeat three times, with a short
rest in between.

*Exercise information kindly supplied by the National Respiratory
Training Centre.*

How can I help myself to breathe more efficiently?

When you suffer from chest problems you may have frightening attacks of breathlessness. Breathing exercises will help you to breathe more efficiently and enable you to control attacks of breathlessness. Breath control is a particularly useful technique for people with COPD; it concentrates on using the lower chest and abdomen, while relaxing the upper chest and shoulders. It will help you to slow down your breathing and reduce any feelings of anxiety. This method of breathing – sometimes known as diaphragmatic breathing – will encourage you to use your

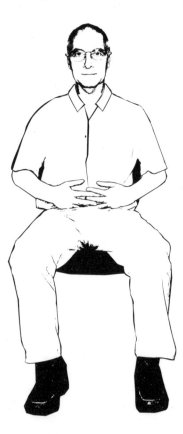

Figure 8.1 The position for practising breathing control.

diaphragm (the main muscle of breathing) more efficiently. You need to concentrate on getting your abdomen to move out as you breathe in rather than allowing it to be sucked inward. Practise breathing control with your hands on your abdomen, as shown in Figure 8.1 and follow the instructions below.

- Sit well supported in an upright position.
- Breathe in deeply to draw air right down to the base of your lungs.
- Breathe out and let the lower ribs sink in as far as possible, pressing gently inwards with your hands at the end of the breath.
- Keep pressing gently and breathe in again, trying to move the lower ribs outwards against your hands.
- Relax, release the pressure and take a normal breath.
- Repeat this exercise five times per session, several times a day.

How can I control my attacks of breathlessness?

Whenever you become breathless, take up one of the positions illustrated below, whichever you find most comfortable. Try to relax and breathe as gently as possible. Breathe at your own rate but, as you gain control, begin to slow the rate of your breathing. Try to use the breathing control technique described in the previous answer.

1 High side lying
This position is particularly useful if you get breathless when lying down. You will need four or five pillows. One pillow should be placed between your waist and armpit; this will keep your back straight and stop you from slipping down the bed. The other pillows are piled up underneath you and the top pillow should be placed above your shoulder to support your head.

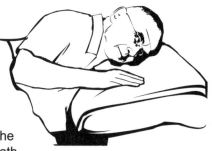

2 Forward lean sitting

You should find this position very relaxing. You will need two or three pillows placed on a table that is high enough for you to rest forward onto.

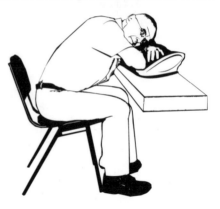

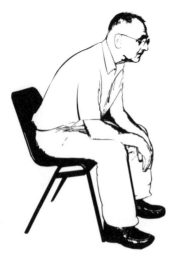

3 Relaxed sitting

You can use this position to rest unobtrusively when you are out, if a seat is available. Sit comfortably, lean forward and rest your forearms along your thighs. Try to keep your back straight, not bent, so that your abdomen can easily move forward when you breathe in.

4 Relaxed standing

You can use this position when you are out and there is no seat available. Stand about a foot from the wall and then lean back gently against it. Try to relax your shoulders and let your arms hang by your sides, or rest your arms on your thighs.

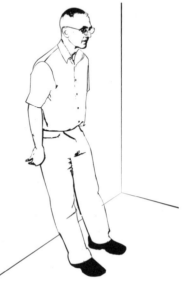

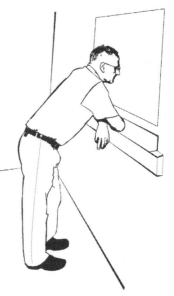

5 Forward-lean stand
Here you just relax, lean forward and
rest your forearms on any stable object
of a suitable height, such as a window-
sill. One of our patients uses this position when he is out shopping, resting on
railings in the local shopping centre. He
just looks as though he is watching the
world go by!

**My father has severe COPD and isn't really able to get
out of the house. Would exercise help him to get fit
enough to get out and about?**

Even small amounts of exercise can be beneficial, so it is worth
your father trying to keep as active as possible. He should be able
to practise breathing control (see the earlier two answers) even
if he finds it difficult to walk or move around. If he is well enough,
he could try adapting some of the exercises illustrated in this
section. Shoulder shrugging, full arm circling, increasing arm
circles, abdominal exercises and quadriceps exercises can all be
done while sitting in a chair. A few of our patients have developed
this routine further to include using light weights. They haven't
gone to great expense, just used a baked bean can in each hand!
Even simple bending and stretching may improve your father's
ability to carry out day-to-day activities.

Your father will probably have good and bad days. When he has
a good day, encourage him to be as active as possible, moving
around from room to room if he can. On bad days he may need to
rest more. He probably has a short-acting beta-2 'reliever' inhaler;

if so, a good tip is to try using it five minutes before attempting an activity – it may help in lessening the breathlessness.

Many doctors now have access to rehabilitation services, including physiotherapy and occupational therapy. If this is available in your father's area, he might be able to have an assessment of his physical ability level to see if this type of service could be of help (see Chapter 9, *Living with COPD*). Encourage your father to have a chat with his doctor or nurse about getting more active.

Is it true that blowing up balloons can help my breathing?

There is some debate as to the benefit of training your breathing muscles, especially those you use when breathing out – as when blowing up balloons. There is even a possibility that this type of blowing exercise may cause problems for some people with certain types of emphysematous bullae (large, cyst-type structures in the lungs). Certainly this type of exercise has been shown to be beneficial in people with no lung disease, so we could suppose that it would be even better with COPD. However, there is very little evidence of this helping people with COPD. It would be best to ask your doctor or nurse for further advice.

I have read about a 'power breathe' device and was wondering if I should buy one for my mum to help her COPD.

The POWERbreathe is a small hand-held device that has been developed to exercise and strengthen muscles involved in breathing in. It uses a technique known as resistance training, in much the same way as you might use weights to increase the strength of your arm muscles. Breathing in through a mouthpiece against resistance, using a little more effort than normal, makes the diaphragm and other muscles involved in breathing work harder, to improve their strength and endurance. The manufacturer recommends that POWERbreathe be used for 30 breaths, twice a day; an improvement should be seen within three to six weeks.

As with all complementary therapies, the POWERbreathe may be used as an adjunct, not alternative, to your mother's regular treatment; it should not replace regular activity and exercise. Your mother should discuss the possible use and safety of this device with her doctor or nurse before you buy it.

I have heard about a device called a 'flutter'. Is it useful in COPD?

The Flutter is a small hand-held device that has been developed to help clear phlegm from the airways. Looking rather like a pipe, the Flutter contains a small ball-bearing in an enclosed compartment. As you breathe out, the ball-bearing vibrates, or *flutters*, creating a slight and changeable resistance in air flow and in air movement. This vibration causes secretions in the airways to loosen, to try to make them easier to cough up. People with cystic fibrosis have used the Flutter with good effect. We have found the Flutter to be useful for people with COPD who produce a lot of phlegm. As with all complementary therapies, the Flutter should be used alongside your regular pre-scribed treatment. If you think the Flutter might benefit you, talk to your doctor or nurse about it.

Pulmonary rehabilitation

The latest Government-backed guidelines from the National Institute for Clinical Excellence (NICE) for the management of COPD suggest that anyone who is 'functionally disabled' by their COPD should be referred to a pulmonary rehabilitation programme. This means that, if your breathlessness is affecting your daily life – having to walk slower, having difficulty walking uphill or climbing stairs, not being able to do your household chores – you would be suitable for pulmonary rehabilitation. A scale that can identify functional disability is the MRC (Medical Research Council) dyspnoea scale, as shown in Table 8.1. If you grade yourself 3 or above, you could benefit from a pulmonary rehabilitation programme.

Table 8.1 MRC dyspnoea scale

Grade	Degree of breathlessness related to activities
1	Not troubled by breathlessness except on strenuous exercise
2	Short of breath when hurrying or walking up a slight hill
3	Walks slower than contemporaries on the level because of breathlessness, or has to stop for breath when walking at own pace
4	Stops for breath after walking about 100 metres or after a few minutes on the level
5	Too breathless to leave the house, or breathless when dressing or undressing

What is pulmonary rehabilitation?

The dictionary definition of rehabilitation is

'to restore to good condition; to make fit after disablement or illness'.

Pulmonary rehabilitation is a medically supervised programme designed to help people with lung disease, including COPD, cope with their illness, restore their ability to function independently and to live the best quality of life they possibly can physically, emotionally and psychologically. Pulmonary rehabilitation can reduce symptoms and improve physical performance to a level better than many drug treatments.

Pulmonary rehabilitation programmes vary in content, length and style but usually involve supervised physical activity (exercise training) combined with an educational content that is based on improving your knowledge of COPD so that you can become more involved in its treatment and management. There may also be the opportunity to talk to counsellors or psychologists so that you can discuss emotional problems, and welfare rights or social workers are often available to offer help with social and financial problems. Courses are run on a group basis that encourages support among its members.

Pulmonary rehabilitation can help you to:

- reduce and control breathing problems,
- become more active,
- stop smoking, and eat healthily and well,
- learn more about the condition and the various treatment options to enable you to develop coping strategies so that you can become more confident and involved in managing your COPD.

I get very breathless when I walk and this can make me feel so anxious that I do not want to go out on my own. My doctor has recommended a pulmonary rehabilitation course – will it help me?

Getting breathless when you walk is a very common symptom of COPD that can cause fear and panic. Be reassured that these are natural feelings. But if you reduce your activity levels, your skeletal muscles will become de-conditioned and this will increase your problems with walking because your legs get tired so easily. We know many people with COPD who avoid any activity that makes them breathless. They tend to lose confidence and become more isolated, not going shopping and not mixing socially, and over time they become increasingly dependent on others to do all the things that they once did themselves. A vicious cycle develops of dependence, disability and worsening quality of life.

It is vital to understand that, although your breathlessness feels very frightening, it is *not* dangerous. In fact, increasing your activity levels can boost your confidence and make you feel less breathless on exertion. Pulmonary rehabilitation will certainly do this by breaking the cycle of decline (Figure 8.2).

I have been referred to a pulmonary rehabilitation programme at the hospital. What should I expect?

Most hospital programmes involve a holistic approach to medical care so you can expect to meet a multi-disciplinary team

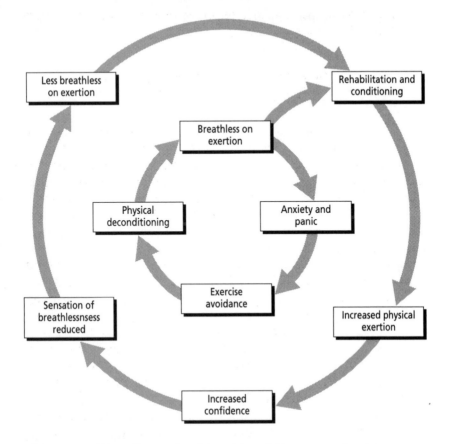

Figure 8.2 The effects of activity or inactivity on exercise tolerance. (Reproduced by permission of the National Respiratory Training Centre.)

including doctors, nurses and physiotherapists. You may also meet occupational therapists, dietitians, social workers and psychologists. A unique programme will be developed to meet your individual needs, and you will attend up to three times a week for 6–12 weeks. Your partner or carer will be actively encouraged to attend as well. Although all programmes vary slightly, you should expect exercise training, education about the disease and its management, and any psychosocial support you require (see details in the next answer).

I am worried about the exercise training part of the pulmonary rehabilitation programme. What will be involved?

As we are sure you have realised by now, exercise, especially aerobic training (the sort that makes you breathe harder) to recondition skeletal muscles and improve your exercise endurance, forms the cornerstone of most pulmonary rehabilitation programmes. The amount of exercise prescribed for you will be determined after an assessment of your individual ability and need. The assessment may involve you walking on a treadmill, or pedalling an exercise bike, or simply performing a shuttle-walking test (see the next answer). Generally, your individual exercise prescription will include a regular form of exercise that you will be able to continue at home, both while you are involved in a rehabilitation programme and after. You may be given a scale to rate your breathlessness on, and you will usually be encouraged to exercise to at least a moderate degree of breathlessness. A scale that is often used for this purpose is known as the Borg Scale, and most people would be encouraged to exercise to between levels 3 and 5 (see Table 8.2).

Exercises that train specific groups of muscles, such as those in your arms, shoulders, back and neck, will usually be included in your training programme. This is because many people with COPD use the muscles in their shoulders, back and neck to help them breathe, so any activity that uses these muscles (e.g. brushing your hair or carrying shopping) is likely to increase the level of your breathlessness. Some centres also include respiratory muscle training to increase strength and endurance, even though this remains an area of controversy.

My doctor mentioned walking tests. What are they?

Walking tests are usually used to judge how far you can walk in a given time, to assess the level and intensity of exercise that will

Table 8.2 The Borg Scale

0	Nothing at all (no breathlessness)
0.5	Very, very slight (just noticeable)
1	Very slight
2	Slight (light)
3	Moderate
4	Somewhat severe
5	Severe (heavy)
6	
7	Very severe
8	
9	
10	Very, very severe (almost maximal)
	Maximal

be suitable for you. They are also useful as a measure of your improvement from pulmonary rehabilitation. There are a number of different tests, and you may be involved with any of them.

- A *six-minute walk* is a standardised test where you will be encouraged to walk as far as possible at your own pace, indoors, on the flat, over a six-minute period. You will be allowed stops if needed, and you will be encouraged to keep going! The total distance you cover in the six minutes is recorded.
- *Shuttle-walking tests* are similar to the six-minute walk, and involve walking between two points for as long as you can at a pace controlled by bleep signals from an audiocassette.
- The *incremental shuttle-walking test* involves you walking between two points, trying to reach one point before a bleep. The bleeps come faster as the test progresses, encouraging you to walk faster in order to assess your maximal exercise capacity.
- The *endurance shuttle-walking test* uses a similar format but measures how long you can maintain your maximal exercise capacity.

Although they may sound daunting, all these tests are done under
supervision so they are really nothing to worry about.

What sorts of things will be covered in the education sessions?

The education sessions will vary from course to course but will
be aimed at helping you and your family to understand COPD, its
treatment and management, and how to live and cope with it.
There will usually be specific sessions covering:

- the lungs in health and disease,
- drug treatments,
- self-management,
- stopping smoking (if appropriate),
- nutrition,
- relaxation and breathing control,
- living and coping with COPD on a daily basis,
- financial support and benefits.

One of the greatest benefits of attending a course is meeting
others with the same condition. You and your partner or carer
will make new friends and benefit from the support of other
group members. The British Lung Foundation's Breathe Easy
groups are often represented at pulmonary rehabilitation
courses; they can provide an ongoing forum for social contact,
support and encouragement that will continue after your course
is over.

I am not sure what all the different people at my pulmonary rehabilitation class do. Can you explain?

You will certainly meet many professionals from both a health
and social care background, and it can be difficult to see where
they all fit in.

- A *chest doctor* will supervise most courses. His or her role
  will be to assess the severity of your COPD and to ensure

that you are having the correct treatment and that the course is suitable and safe for you. The doctor may also be involved in some of the education sessions.

- A *specialist respiratory nurse* is often involved in supervising the course, delivering the education sessions, participating in or supervising exercise sessions. He or she may also be your first point of contact for information, help and advice.
- *Physiotherapists* often supervise the exercise sessions. They can teach breathing control and relaxation exercises. They can also be of great help to people who have problems with phlegm clearance.
- *Dietitians* can provide valuable advice on healthy eating; they will also be available to provide specific advice to anyone who is underweight or overweight.
- *Occupational therapists* are there to help you make the most of your abilities, despite your breathlessness, by giving you specific exercises and providing specialist equipment to help you improve your ability to care for yourself. They will usually do a detailed assessment of what your problems are and will give advice on and provide any equipment that will make your life easier.
- The *social worker* will be able to give advice on benefits and financial matters; they can also help with housing and general social care issues – for example, home help support and meals-on-wheels.
- Some programmes also have the support of a *counsellor* or *clinical psychologist* who can help with anxiety, depression, and marital and sexual problems.
- Most programmes will have access to a specialist *smoking-cessation adviser*, if needed.

My GP practice is starting a pulmonary rehabilitation course. Will it be as effective as the hospital courses?

Because of the relative scarcity of pulmonary rehabilitation courses, a few GP practices and primary care organisations are looking to develop courses in their local area. This is quite a new development so we don't have any personal experience of it but there is some research to suggest that you should do just as well so long as all the recommended elements (see the answers above) are included. It isn't where the course is run, or who runs it, rather what it consists of that is the most crucial element. Good luck and enjoy it!

Why isn't there a pulmonary rehabilitation course in my local area?

This is a difficult one to answer. Most chest doctors believe that pulmonary rehabilitation is a very effective form of treatment that can improve exercise tolerance and quality of life for people with COPD. A major difficulty is lack of funds and staff to run regular courses. The good news is that more hospitals are setting up courses every year, and alternative venues and sources of funding are being sought: for example, some primary care trusts and individual GP surgeries are developing courses at a local level (which will mean less travelling for the patients). The bottom line, however, is that, unless people with COPD demand this form of treatment, additional funding will not be made available. So our advice is to start asking questions of the senior people at the hospital and the primary care organisation, and your MP, too.

I have quite mild COPD; will I be able to get onto a pulmonary rehabilitation course?

At the present time, because they are in such short supply, most hospital courses are open only to people with moderate and severe COPD; this is not to say you would not be accepted, but it is usually only those with moderate and severe disease who are referred to the hospital! You need to discuss a referral with your doctor. If the availability of courses becomes more widespread, this sort of policy may change.

The best thing you can do until this happens is to get as active as you can. Ask your doctor or nurse if there is an 'exercise on prescription' scheme in your area. Check out what is available at local leisure centres. Many gyms and leisure centres hold special classes for over-50s, which may be especially suitable; don't feel that you have to go out and buy all the latest equipment. If none of these suits you or your lifestyle, just try to get out for a regular walk, increase your activity level at home and practise some of the simple exercises given earlier in this chapter.

I feel so much better since going on the pulmonary rehabilitation course. How can I keep myself feeling fit and active?

The benefits of your course will be long lasting but cannot persist forever if you stop your exercise and activity programme. It can be difficult to keep up with the programme once you are away from the support of your group but maintaining your improvement depends on your self-reliance and motivation to continue. Some centres offer occasional refresher sessions or provide a 'training diary' of exercise and activity for you to follow. In others, patient support groups continue to provide the motivation. The ideal may be to graduate from your course to an alternative exercise programme at a local gym or leisure centre where you can continue to meet regularly, exercise and benefit from mutual support.

9
Living with COPD

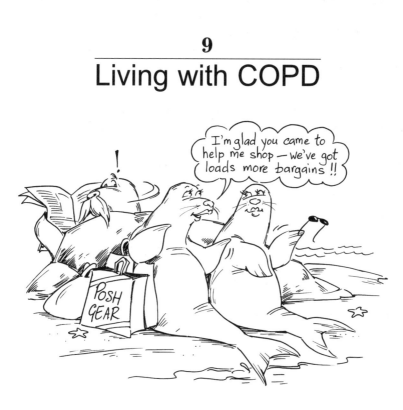

Helping yourself

There are a number of things that you can do to help yourself overcome the problems associated with COPD, and prevent deterioration in your condition.

- Stop smoking.
- Keep as active as possible.
- Maintain your weight at a sensible level and eat a healthy diet.
- Have a flu vaccination every year.

- Ask your GP for a pneumonia vaccination.
- Take simple measures to try to avoid chest infections.
- Be able to recognise when your condition is worsening and take appropriate action.

These points are discussed in more detail below.

STOPPING SMOKING

Do I really need to stop smoking?

If you are really serious about helping yourself, you need to do whatever you can to prevent your COPD from getting worse. Stopping smoking is the most important thing you can do. There has never been a better time to stop smoking. Have a look at Chapter 4, *Stopping smoking*, for more help and advice.

KEEPING ACTIVE

I get short of breath when I am out shopping. Is this dangerous?

It is natural to assume that breathlessness is dangerous. However, the breathlessness associated with activity in COPD is not dangerous and will not cause further lung damage although it can cause you to worry and feel anxious. If you start to avoid activity, you will become unfit and your muscles will get de-conditioned, and this will lead in turn to leg tiredness, which can stop you walking. You may also lose confidence in your ability to go shopping on your own.

The best thing you can do is continue to be as active as possible. Your doctor or nurse should be able to increase or change your medication to help you manage your breathlessness more successfully, and you can learn simple techniques to help you control your breathing more effectively. You can find more detail about exercise and fitness in Chapter 8.

Would it be OK for me to join a gym and take up some regular exercise?

What a positive idea! Taking up regular exercise will improve your general fitness, reduce your overall sensation of breathlessness and increase your confidence. Although having COPD alone should not prevent you from joining a gym, we would advise you to have a chat with your doctor or nurse beforehand to ensure that you are OK. They will also be able to adjust your medication if necessary to help reduce breathlessness.

Do I have to join a gym to get fit?

Some form of regular exercise will have benefits for most people with COPD; whether this is at a gym or at home is merely personal preference. Walking and stair climbing would both fit in with your everyday life and you might be more likely to stick with these activities on a regular basis. Some of our patients have had great success improving their general fitness through gentle exercise such as walking rather than joining a gym.

If you want to join a gym but are worried about the cost, ask your GP if the practice has access to a supervised exercise programme at a local leisure centre. This scheme, often known as 'exercise on prescription' is not available everywhere but it would certainly be worthwhile contacting your GP surgery to see what is on hand locally. The fees for this sort of exercise programme vary from area to area but they are usually nominal.

Are there any exercises I can do at home?

There are indeed some exercises that you can do at home that will improve your general fitness. Details of these can be found in Chapter 8 (*Exercise and fitness*). The British Lung Foundation produces some excellent leaflets containing information about suitable gentle exercise and breathing control. Their contact details are in the Appendix (*Useful addresses*).

MAINTAIN A NORMAL BODY WEIGHT

My GP has asked me to try to lose some weight. Can you help?

Being overweight adds to your breathlessness. Carrying too much weight increases your body's need for oxygen to enable you to carry out any exercise or day-to-day activity. Your lungs are not able to expand as effectively, thus increasing the work of breathing, and your heart is also under extra strain. So anything you can do to get some weight off will help your breathlessness.

To lose some weight you need to control your calorie intake, eat a healthy balance of foods and increase your exercise level if possible. Try to lose the excess weight slowly, 1 to 2 pounds a week is recommended. Do not go on a crash diet – they leave you feeing tired and run down, and you'll probably soon put back all the weight you lost. Top tips include:

- Grill rather than fry food.
- Cut all visible fat off meat before cooking.
- Eat at least five portions of fruit and vegetables a day.
- Cut down on all fats such as butter and cheese, and don't forget the hidden fat in cakes, biscuits and pastry.
- Limit your alcohol intake.
- Chew your food slowly.

If you are struggling, your GP or practice nurse may be able to offer extra support and motivation, and can refer you to a dietitian if necessary.

My father has severe COPD and has started to lose weight. What can I do?

Many people with severe COPD are either underweight or start to lose weight as time goes by. It is thought that weight loss occurs through the excessive use of energy by overworked respiratory muscles and the changes that occur in the body due to lack of oxygen.

As breathing can be very hard work, your father may have problems with loss of appetite, early fullness, bloating and increased breathlessness during and after eating. Supplementing his diet with extra food may increase these problems. There are several things you could try to halt your father's weight loss.

- Encourage your father to try smaller meals more often. Six small meals a day will make him less breathless than three larger ones.
- If chewing food tires him out, try liquidising it, or making home-made soup, home-made milk shakes and milky drinks. Commercial products such as Build Up and Complan may help.
- Go for high-energy food. This advice may go against what you know about healthy eating, but if your father stops eating he will not be able to maintain his weight and he will deteriorate further. So go for full fat milk, cream and butter!
- Avoid bulky, gassy foods that cause bloating. Distension of the stomach will press on the lungs and cause increased breathlessness. Among the worst offenders are peas and beans, cabbage and sprouts.
- Avoid hard, dry foods such as crackers that need a lot of chewing. Go for soft foods and add liquid such as custard, gravy or a sauce.
- Your father's GP can arrange for a nutritional assessment and can provide supplements on prescription if needed. He or she may also consider referral to a dietitian.

I have read that I should take extra vitamins for my COPD. Is this true?

There is some research evidence to suggest that vitamin C deficiency may be linked to the development of COPD, and that a high intake of vitamin C is associated with better lung function. Although in these studies people who ate little fruit tended to have an unhealthy lifestyle (taking little exercise, smoking or living with a smoker, and living in an urban area), this did not seem to be an explanation for the differences. The difference between those who ate fresh fruit more than once a day and those who ate fresh fruit less than once a week was equivalent to the adverse effects of smoking 20 cigarettes a day for between seven and ten years.

The reason for this difference is unclear, although it is thought that vitamin C may protect against the destructive effects of tobacco smoke, reduce inflammation and promote lung growth and repair. So eating fresh fruit more than once a day may be better than taking vitamin supplements.

AVOID INFECTIONS

My doctor says I need a flu vaccination every year. Why is this – I thought it was only necessary for elderly people?

The Department of Health recommends that everyone over the age of 65 years be vaccinated against flu every year. It is also recommended for people with a range of chronic diseases, including COPD. Flu vaccination has reduced the number of deaths, serious illness and complications following flu among the elderly by 70 per cent. Because having COPD makes you more prone to the complications of flu, there ought to be benefits from annual flu vaccination.

The vaccination has to be given every year because the flu virus itself changes regularly and our bodies need to be primed to fight off the current version. Every year the World Health Organization tries to predict which type of flu virus will circulate, and this information is passed to the manufacturers who attempt to produce and deliver the vaccine by September/October each year. Flu is most prevalent from around mid-December so it is a good idea to get your jab early. Most GP practices hold flu clinics every October/November, so don't ignore your invitation letter or the posters and advertisements; be sure to make an appointment.

My GP wants me to have a flu vaccination. Will it give me flu?

Because the flu vaccination does not contain the live virus, it cannot give you flu, but it won't prevent you from getting a cold either. As colds are prevalent at the same time that the flu jab is given, many people confuse the two. The vaccine makes your body produce antibodies against the flu virus and this process can cause a few minor transient symptoms such as headache and fever. But these symptoms are nothing like the flu that will make you feel so unwell that it is difficult to get out of bed. Anyone who has had influenza will know the difference between a cold and true flu! The flu virus (not the vaccination) is also known to be associated with severe chest infections and pneumonia. Our advice would be to discuss any worries with your doctor or nurse.

When I went for my flu jab the practice nurse offered me vaccination against pneumonia as well. What is this jab and should I have it done?

This vaccination provides protection against the most common cause of pneumonia in the community – pneumococcal pneumonia. This type of infection is more common in adults over 50 years of age, and vaccination is recommended by the Department of Health for people with COPD. For most people this is a single injection that will offer life-long protection. There are a few conditions, such as low immunity, that warrant vaccination every five years. Low immunity is not a common condition but a few people with COPD will have it; if you do, you will usually have been told about this and given advice about vaccinations. If you are unsure, your GP or practice nurse will be able to offer further advice.

We have found that this vaccine is very well tolerated and can be given safely at the same time as the flu jab (but in the other arm). Like the flu jab, it can give you a few minor symptoms such as headache for a couple of days but the benefit of reduced risk of pneumonia should outweigh this.

Should I try to avoid catching a cold?

Bouts of bronchitis often follow a cold, and some people with COPD seem to suffer more than others. Colds are viruses that infect the throat and nose and give symptoms for up to a week but usually without complications. However, if you have COPD a simple cold can leave your airways more prone to secondary bacterial infection that quickly turns into a chest infection. The medical terminology for this is 'an acute exacerbation of COPD' (see also the next answer). Keeping clear of colds is not easy but if you can avoid people who are coughing and sneezing, your risk of infection will fall. It is probably worth discussing this with family and friends, who should postpone visiting you if they have a cold. Prompt treatment of an exacerbation of your COPD will mean that you do not get as ill, that you get better faster and that you can reduce your risk of having to be admitted to hospital.

RECOGNISING AND MANAGING ACUTE EXACERBATIONS OF COPD

How can I recognise an acute exacerbation of COPD?

Many of you will readily recognise the signs of an acute exacerbation, but it has taken a while for doctors and nurses to realise that you do! The key signs are:

- increasing breathlessness, wheeze and chest tightness,
- increasing phlegm production,
- a change in the colour of your phlegm from white or clear to green or yellow.

You may also feel hot and sweaty, weak and tired, and cannot stop coughing. Sometimes, especially if your COPD is severe, you may develop fluid retention and ankle swelling; always see your GP if this happens.

Prompt treatment of these symptoms is very important but many of you will find that you cannot get an appointment to see your GP straight away. For this reason it is a good idea for you to be able to recognise the signs and to be able to take action yourself. Increasingly, people with COPD are being issued with the resources to start treatment themselves. We call this self-management. Many doctors now prefer to give prescriptions in advance, so that you can get them filled and start treatment as soon as you feel unwell. People with severe COPD may have direct access to the respiratory nurse specialist or hospital ward.

All this saves valuable time, and can reduce the severity, and
shorten the duration, of the exacerbation.

How is an acute exacerbation treated?

The vast majority of exacerbations respond well to antibiotic
treatment. You should notice an improvement within 48 hours.
If you are not starting to improve, or your condition is worsening, or if your breathlessness has worsened so that it is affecting your normal activities, you should seek further advice from
your GP.

Sometimes you will also be prescribed a short course (one to
two weeks) of oral steroids to reduce inflammation in your chest.
This is usually done if you have severe COPD, if you have some
asthma, or if you are failing to get better on antibiotics alone. If
you are more breathless or wheezy, it is also recommended that
you start (or increase) your bronchodilator treatment or use your
nebuliser if you have one. Your doctor or nurse will advise you.

Although most people will respond well to this treatment, a
small number will need specialist attention from the hospital,
where their condition will be thoroughly assessed. They will have
a chest x-ray and some blood tests, and further treatment will be
started as necessary. An increasing number of hospitals now
offer the choice of being admitted to the ward or being cared for
by a specialist team at home – if this is appropriate.

What is 'hospital at home'?

Basically, it means receiving hospital-type treatment at home.
There is a growing trend for people with severe acute exacerbations of their COPD to be admitted to a hospital assessment unit.
If they are found to be suitable, they will be returned home to be
cared for by a specialist respiratory nurse who visits daily until
they are recovered or, if their condition deteriorates, will readmit
them to hospital. This type of service is known as the Acute
Respiratory Assessment Service or ARAS.

Other hospitals have an early-discharge scheme whereby the
person is admitted to a hospital ward and then discharged home

early if appropriate, with the support of a specialist respiratory nurse.

Most people are very satisfied with being treated at home by a specialist nurse, and research shows that they do just as well as those who have been admitted to hospital.

In some areas there is also a 'rapid response' team (nurses, physiotherapist, occupational therapist) who can assess, treat and manage people in their own homes to help them get over an acute illness. This level of care can only be provided in the short term – up to two weeks – but it can prevent the need for admission to hospital.

I live quite a distance from my mum, who is in hospital following a severe exacerbation of her COPD. She has been very unwell and I don't think she will be able to cope at home on her own yet. I have heard there is an intermediate care team who will help. Can you tell me more?

'Intermediate care' is a service that bridges the gap between hospital and home, and there are a growing number of intermediate care teams across the UK. There are different types and levels of support, which includes nursing, rehabilitation services and social care. The team is made up of doctors, nurses, physiotherapists, occupational therapists, social workers and care workers.

The usual procedure would be that, when your mum is well enough, she would have a full assessment of her needs, and the level and type of care required would then be then put in place. She might be offered a short-term stay in a rehabilitation unit, or given care and support at home. Speak to the hospital social worker for more detailed information about what is available in her area.

I am very unhappy with the care I am receiving. Whom can I talk to about this?

In the first instance, it is usually best to sit down and discuss any problems with the individuals concerned. Putting your thoughts down on paper can help you clarify the main issues.

If your problems are not resolved, the next step would be to approach an advocacy service. This type of advocacy used to be provided by the local Community Health Council (CHC); however, these are being abolished and replaced by a couple of alternatives.

The Patient Advocacy and Liaison Service (PALS) has been set up in each primary care trust (PCT) and hospital. Its duties are to:

- provide information about local health services and local support groups;
- provide information on complaints procedures and act as a gateway to the Independent Complaints and Advocacy Service (ICAS);
- resolve problems on the spot, if possible;
- act as an early-warning system to the PCTs and hospitals by reporting gaps in the health service as they become aware of them.

The Independent Complaints and Advocacy Service is responsible for arranging advocacy services for patients wishing to make a formal complaint against the NHS.

Holidays and travel

Holidays provide a change of scene and a change from the routine of daily life. If you have COPD, this can pose a number of problems. Before you go away on holiday, it would be sensible to have a chat with your doctor or nurse about your fitness to travel to certain destinations. Always get advice about your medical fitness to travel if you have severe COPD, or have been in hospital with an exacerbation in the last year or you are using oxygen at home. You should also consider, well in advance, where you want to go (the UK or abroad?), any equipment you will need, whether the terrain will be hilly or flat, and how you will get there.

My husband and I used to go abroad for our holidays but now I have been told I have COPD. Can you give me some general advice about travelling outside the UK?

You should be able to continue as normal but it is best to be prepared. First, think ahead. Be sure to leave plenty of time to plan what you will need; don't leave anything to the last minute. Think about what you must take with you. Choose a holiday that you can cope with now, not one you enjoyed in the past. Think about your destination: what are the facilities like, will there be stairs to climb, is the terrain hilly, will there be transport that you can use without difficulty?

Don't forget that you may need to be vaccinated against certain diseases before you travel to more exotic destinations; having COPD does not change this advice. You should contact your GP surgery six to eight weeks in advance to find out about vaccination for travel. *Health Advice for Travellers* is a booklet from the Department of Health, containing comprehensive information about health risks, health-care costs and the vaccination requirements for different countries.

It might be a good idea to make an appointment to see your GP or practice nurse for a check-up before you travel. To avoid any last-minute problems, this should also be one to two weeks before you leave. At this appointment, ask your GP or nurse to provide you with antibiotics (and steroid tablets if appropriate) to use in case you have an acute exacerbation of COPD while you are away. Order all the medication you will need while away at least a week in advance.

Make sure you pack your medication in your hand luggage, not in your suitcase, in case you need to use an inhaler on the aircraft (or in case your luggage gets lost!). Check out the availability of medical services in the resort you are travelling to – if not before you go, then on arrival at your destination.

Follow all the usual travel advice:

- Use a high factor sun-screen.
- Don't drink the local water in developing countries; boil the water or buy bottled water (perhaps get fizzy water, as it has been known for bottles to be filled with ordinary tap

water and sold as still mineral water).

- Avoid salads unless you have washed them yourself, and don't have ice cubes unless you have made them from bottled water.
- Avoid ice-cream from street vendors.
- Make sure you have adequate holiday insurance.

Will having COPD affect my travel insurance?

As for anyone going away on holiday (or on business, for that matter), having full travel insurance is a must. The standard premium will usually require that you are completely fit and healthy, and some companies will not accept people who have significant health problems. Shop around for a company that will give you appropriate cover, in the knowledge that you have COPD.

The British Lung Foundation can give you more help and advice on this matter.

What is the European Health Insurance Card?

A European Health Insurance Card (EHIC) entitles you to reduced-cost, sometimes free, medical treatment while you are in a European Economic Area (EEA) country or Switzerland. The EEA consists of the European Union (EU) countries plus Iceland, Liechtenstein and Norway.

The EHIC has replaced the old E111, which was withdrawn on 1 January 2006. You can apply for an EHIC by completing a form obtainable from the post office or online at the Department of Health website. You can also apply by telephone on 0845 606 2030; you will need to provide your name, date of birth and NHS or National Insurance number, so have this information to hand.

The EHIC is normally valid for three to five years and covers any medical treatment that becomes necessary during your trip, because of either illness or an accident. The card gives you access to state-provided medical treatment only, and you'll be treated on the same basis as an 'insured' person living in the country you're visiting. Note that this might not cover all the things you'd expect to get free of charge from the NHS in the UK. You might have to make a contribution to the cost of your care.

The EHIC also covers any treatment you need for a chronic disease or pre-existing illness. You must make arrangements in advance for oxygen therapy. We strongly advise that you discuss your travel plans with your specialist oxygen team before you make any arrangements. Some limited information on oxygen supply services in the EEA countries and Switzerland is available from the Department of Health's Customer Service Centre (see Appendix 1 for their telephone number).

I have stable but severe COPD and want to visit my daughter in the USA. Will I have any problems?

You need to discuss this with your doctor before you make any travel plans that include flying. The cabin pressures in an aircraft are equivalent to being at the top of a mountain 5,000–8,000 feet above sea level where the air is thin and has less oxygen. This means that the air you breathe when flying contains 15–16 per cent oxygen rather than the 21 per cent you are used to breathing on the ground. Normally this would not be a problem, but with severe COPD the low level of oxygen in the air can cause a potentially hazardous fall in the oxygen level in your blood.

In deciding whether they can safely accept someone as a passenger, airlines often use the criterion of the person being able to walk for 50 yards without breathlessness. If they cannot achieve this, it indicates a need for further investigation. The further investigations will usually be done at the hospital but, because not all hospitals have the facilities to carry out the assessments, you might have to travel to one that does. The assessments will include measuring lung function and doing blood tests to measure both oxygen and carbon dioxide levels.

If you require supplementary oxygen, it can be arranged on most scheduled flights. Approach the airline well in advance, giving them information about your oxygen requirements. The cost of providing this can vary from nothing to £100, depending on the airline, so shop around! Or contact the British Lung Foundation for their information.

Remember to inform the airline if you will need a wheelchair or other help at the airport. If you use a nebuliser, you may have to use it during the flight because the atmosphere in the plane will be dry and will tend to dry your secretions. There should be no problem with these issues provided you let the airline know about them well in advance.

I am on long-term oxygen therapy for COPD. Can I still travel abroad?

It may be possible to do this but you should check with your doctor that you are fit enough – and it will take a great deal of planning. You will need to check that oxygen is available for your journey and at your destination. It would be wise to find out where the local hospital or clinic is situated – and if it has the facilities to treat any problems that may arise while you are there. You will most likely also have to pay for some of these services, including oxygen when abroad.

You need enough medication for your journey (remember to keep it in your hand luggage) and for the time you are away – plus any additional treatment such as antibiotics and steroid tablets in case you have an exacerbation. Don't forget spare filters and masks or mouthpieces for your nebuliser if you have one – and check in advance that it will run on the local power supply.

You will also need to think about how you get around – do you need a wheelchair and assistance during transit? Your choice of destination will also be important – a hilly resort any distance from medical services would not be suitable! Travel insurance is likely to require a higher premium, and airlines and ferries for example may make a charge for providing or transporting additional oxygen – so it could be an expensive trip!

All this will take careful planning well in advance of travel and will involve a great deal of checking to make sure that everything is in place. If you decide to go ahead, have a good holiday!

I have emphysema and have been told that I should not fly. Why is this?

Not everyone with emphysema is given this advice, so we suspect that you probably have something known as *emphysematous bullae*. Bullae are formed when the walls of the alveoli (the tiny sacs in the lungs where gas exchange takes place) are destroyed.

Alveoli are normally packed together like a bunch of grapes but when their walls are destroyed, the 'bunch of grapes' is destroyed and a larger balloon-like structure is formed – a bulla. These balloon-like structures in the chest can expand as the cabin pressure falls, compressing the rest of the lung. In severe cases there is a risk that a bulla can 'burst' and cause air leakage from the lungs into the surrounding tissues. This is known as a *pneumothorax* and is a medical emergency. This is why, for you, travel by land or sea will be less hazardous.

Will flying affect my inhalers?

Flying will not adversely affect your inhalers, even your pressurised metered-dose inhaler. Although airline regulations state that you should not carry pressurised canisters in your hand luggage, the airlines recognise that people with COPD do need to carry their inhalers with them. It is better to carry your inhalers in your hand luggage so that you have your treatment to hand if you need it.

It is safe to use all forms of inhalers during your flight. However, a pressurised inhaler will need to be at room temperature when you use it. If it feels cold to the touch, warm it in your hands before use. Dry power inhalers such as Accuhaler, Turbohaler and HandiHaler are not affected by temperature.

My father is on long-term oxygen and I want to take him to the seaside for a week this summer. How can I do this?

This should be a fairly easy task so long as you plan ahead. The oxygen concentrator can be unplugged, put in the boot of your car and plugged in again when you arrive at your destination. However, you should check that your insurance will cover this. Your home oxygen supply company can arrange to deliver an oxygen concentrator to your holiday destination. They need around four weeks' notice to be able to do this. Be sure to let your GP or practice nurse know well in advance – they will complete a holiday Home Oxygen Order Form (HOOF) and inform the oxygen supply company, who will then arrange delivery. If you need portable oxygen for the journey or to use when out and about, this can be arranged at the same time.

Many hotels and guest-houses have facilities for disabled people and ground-floor rooms, which will make it easier for your father to move around. Tourism for All National Accessible Accommodation Standards (TANAAS) assesses the accessibility of all accommodation, including self-catering. The three categories are:

- Category one: accessible to a wheelchair user travelling independently;
- Category two: accessible to a wheelchair user travelling with assistance;
- Category three: accessible to someone with limited mobility but able to walk a few paces and up the maximum three steps.

The Holiday Care Service and the local tourist boards inspect this standard, so, for further information about suitable places to stay, contact the local tourist information service where you would like to stay.

Make sure that your father has enough medication for the duration of the trip plus a bit extra to cover any delays, and that it is easy to access en route. Ask your father's GP for advice about what to do if the symptoms get worse while you are away. If your father has a self-management plan, ensure that he has his emergency treatment with him. Get the telephone numbers of a local GP and hospital in the area you are visiting, just in case you run into any problems. If you do all this well in advance, both you and your father should be able to relax and enjoy your holiday.

I have COPD and want to visit my sister. I can get there by coach or by rail – will there be any problems travelling by either of these means?

If you decide to go by coach, discuss what you will need when you are booking. You may have to contact the coach company and inform them of your travel requirements. Coach journeys can take longer but usually make frequent stops. National Express coaches have 'kneeling suspension', which makes it easier to get on and off. Most of their on-board facilities are on a level with the seating, so there should be no need to use stairs to get to the toilet. Most bus and coach companies will carry lightweight folding wheelchairs.

National Express does not carry batter-powered wheelchairs.

The different rail companies have different policies regarding people with disabilities, so plan your route accordingly. The National Rail Enquiries (08457 48 49 50) will advise you further. All rail companies offer assistance to people who pre-book. Contact the relevant train company and tell them where and when you are travelling, your disability, and how you intend to get to and from the stations. Let them know whether you are travelling alone and if you use a wheelchair. The leaflet *Rail Travel for Disabled Passengers* (available from most staffed railway stations) has helpful advice and outlines the minimum level of service you can expect throughout the UK's rail network.

Learning to pace yourself

Many people with COPD consider that learning to pace themselves was one of the most important things they had to learn after they were diagnosed. Energy is like money in the bank – to be spent wisely. Your limits in coping with daily activities will fluctuate from day to day, or even from hour to hour. Some days you will wake up feeling great and on other days you will know almost immediately that it is a day for resting. It is important to learn to trust these feelings.

I'm having to find ways to pace myself, now that I've been diagnosed with COPD. Have you any tips that would help?

A major factor to bear in mind is never to take on more than you can handle comfortably when you feel tired: build in rest periods or break down a big job into smaller parts. Save certain tasks for good days. When you want to expend more energy than usual, plan for it and use common sense. The suggestions below should help.

- Take your reliever inhaler before you attempt an activity, as you are more likely to be at your best soon after this.
- Do not rush.
- Break big jobs down into smaller parts.
- Wait an hour or more after eating. Digestion draws blood

and oxygen away from muscles, leaving them less able to cope. Also, a full stomach presses up towards your chest, making it harder for your lungs to expand.

- If you feel breathless, stop, rest, relax and use breathing control (see Chapter 8, *Exercise and fitness*).
- Try to keep everything – especially your living area – tidy. Staying on top of things will make your life easier.
- When carrying things upstairs, rest every two or three steps. It may take you longer but it will be possible to get the job done without exhausting yourself. Have a chair to sit on or a table to lean on when you reach the top.
- If you struggle carrying things from room to room, get hold of a lightweight trolley: you can use it to transfer items from one place to another.

Mum is finding that getting dressed in the morning is a great struggle. Can you help?

Most people like to wash and dress before breakfast but if your mum is finding this an effort, she could split the activity into two blocks: wash before breakfast and dress after.

Although what your mum wears should be down to her personal taste, she should consider the type of clothes she is wearing. Fortunately, modern fabrics and styles should mean that your mum does not have to sacrifice style for comfort. Tight bras, corsets or girdles are difficult to put on, and also restrict the chest and abdomen, making breathing even harder, so are best avoided. Cotton camisoles are a comfortable substitute but, if your mum prefers to wear a bra, a sports bra will offer firm but soft support. Trousers and socks are easier to put on than tights. Slip-on shoes are a good choice, too; laces and buckles mean bending over to fasten them, an activity that many people find exhausting. Putting on any kind of shoe is much easier with a long-handled shoe-horn.

We're thinking of getting Mum some aids to help her to get about. How can we find out what's available?

It is part of the role of occupational therapists to provide advice about aids, equipment and assistance with various aspects of daily living to help people function as well as possible. They usually have access to a wide range of equipment that people can try before hiring or buying. They also have catalogues of companies that specialise in providing such aids. Your mum's doctor or nurse can refer you to the occupational therapist. Even if they cannot supply you with an item on the NHS, they will be able to advise you on which items are worth investing in and where you can obtain them. Some towns have shops or showrooms displaying the equipment for you to try out on the premises. The Disabled Living Centres Council (address in the Appendix) can tell you about a centre near you or your mum.

My mother needs a wheelchair to get out and about. The occupational therapist has ordered one but it will be several weeks before it arrives. What can we do in the meantime?

The local branch of the Red Cross will usually be able to rent you one for a small fee. Their number will be listed in the telephone directory.

There are also an increasing number of shops appearing all over the UK that sell and hire equipment for disabled people. Most will hire wheelchairs by the day, week or month. It costs from about £10 per week to hire a lightweight folding wheelchair, plus a refundable deposit.

Dad has COPD and has to go everywhere by car. Can I apply for a Blue Badge for him?

The Blue Badge scheme (replacing the Orange Badge scheme) provides parking concessions for people with severe walking difficulties who travel by car either as drivers or as passengers. Badge holders may park close to their destination but only for on-street parking, and time limits vary from area to area.

There are rules about who can have a badge but your father should qualify. If he has a permanent and substantial disability that results in his being unable to walk or having considerable difficulty in walking, he should be able to get one. You (or he) will need to answer some questions about the level of your father's disability to help the local authority determine whether he is eligible. Applications should be made to the social services department of the local authority (in Scotland, the chief executive or social work department of the local council).

The Blue Badge is a two-sided card with space for a photograph of the badge holder on the back. Your father's application should therefore be accompanied by two recent passport-sized photos, which should be signed on the back. Badges last for three years, and he will need to reapply before his badge expires. For more information, contact your local authority.

I am struggling with having a bath. Do you have any suggestions?

Washing and bathing can use a great deal of energy. You should be able to access aids and adaptations from social services through your GP, nurse, social worker or occupational therapist. Sadly, though, there is often a long wait because of high demand. If you can't wait very long, you can buy many bathing aids from local suppliers or (making sure that you are dealing with a legitimate company) via the Internet. But get professional advice about what aids to buy before laying out any money.

If you find using a shower or bath too demanding, try a bath seat. Bath seats are waterproof and go directly into the bath; they can be removed easily when others want to use the bath. A lightweight hand-spray attached to the bath taps can make hair washing and rinsing less of a chore. If you have a shower cubicle, place a waterproof chair inside to sit on – a plastic garden chair would do; you can buy rubberised pads from a DIY store to place on the base of the legs, to reduce the risk of the chair slipping.

It is not necessary to get wet all over to be clean. A 'basin bath' can be a lot less taxing, especially if you are having a bad day. A long towelling robe will eliminate the effort of drying altogether, just blot.

Remember to sit to dry yourself, shave, apply make-up or dry your hair. Leave the bathroom door slightly ajar or turn on the extractor fan if you have one, to reduce the level of humidity. If you feel weak or are having a bad day, don't take a bath or shower if you are on your own.

**How can I make it easier for my dad to take his
medication – including his nebulised therapy – every day?**

Most pharmacies can supply tablets in weekly blister packs. There
is usually a small charge for this. The alternative is to buy a 'dosette'
box: this is a container with compartments labelled Monday to
Sunday, into which you can place your father's tablets into the
required number of times a day (e.g. morning, midday and evening).
Make sure that he has enough medicines for a week's reserve but
don't order more than he needs, or he might become overloaded
with boxes of tablets and inhalers, which can lead to confusion.

Try to get all your father's nebulising equipment and drugs
together in a convenient place where it can be left between treatments. Being near the kitchen or bathroom, where it is easy to
rinse and clean the nebuliser chamber between use, could be
useful but, if your dad needs to use it at night, you may have to
consider keeping the equipment by his bed. An excellent way to
store spare filters, nebulising chambers and tubing is in plastic
storage boxes.

**I'm beginning to find doing the shopping rather a
struggle. What can I do?**

First try going shopping on quiet days and quiet times. This way
you will be able to move at a leisurely pace and avoid being
jostled. At the supermarket, choose one of the small trolleys;
the big, deep ones make life more difficult as you have to bend
to put items in and then take them out. If your partner or a
friend cannot go with you to help with items on high or low
shelves, ask an assistant for help. Some supermarkets provide
a shopping assistant as a service to customers. Have all your
'spoilable' items, such as fresh or frozen foods, packed in separate bags. When you get home, you can easily identify the
items that need to be put away immediately in the fridge or
freezer and leave the rest for later when you have more energy
or a helper can lend a hand.

Shopping for clothing can be exhausting, even for people in the
best of health! Know your measurements, write them down, and
take a tape measure with you. This may avoid your having to try

on items in the shop. Shop at stores that will allow you to return any item that, when you try it on at home, you realise is not really suitable.

Other possibilities are shopping by mail order and via the Internet, making it unnecessary for you to go out if you don't want to.

Work and employment

Do I have to tell my employer that I have been diagnosed as having COPD?

There is no need to tell anyone at work, unless your condition affects your ability to do your job.

If, however, you are applying for a new job, you may be asked about your health record. If you do not tell the truth then and you get the job, any contract of employment would not be valid and you would have no protection in the event of dismissal.

What are my legal rights? I'm worried that my workplace will get rid of me because of my COPD. I have to lift heavy boxes, which makes me very breathless, but I can cope with the other parts of my job.

This involves the Disability Discrimination Act, a relatively new piece of legislation that applies to larger employers (those with 20 or more employees). In brief, employers are obliged to make 'reasonable' adjustments to the workplace on behalf of their employees with a disability. For example, adjustments may need to be made to someone's work station.

Occupational health doctors are expert in interpreting this new law and making recommendations. For example, a factory worker who had difficulty walking had his workbench placed nearer the lavatory so that he didn't have so far to walk to it. Quite simple changes and adjustments of this sort can help keep people employed and workplaces productive. That's the point of this legislation.

I am sure my employer is trying to ease me out of my job as a warehouseman. I recently had 10 days off work with an infection related to my COPD but I have not had any time off before that. Can I be made to leave work?

Your employer cannot make you leave your job just because you have COPD. Look at your contract of employment to establish what you are entitled to in terms of sick pay. The Disability Discrimination Act 1995 protects your rights if you are working for a company that employs 20 or more people. Employment law is very complicated, so it would be best to seek further advice from your union, Citizens Advice Bureau or other advisory service. The following information may also be useful:

- Since 1999, employers have been obliged to make reasonable adjustments to the workplace or working conditions to make it possible for a person to continue in that job or another within the same company.
- If you want to continue working, your condition alone is not a reason for your company terminating your employment. If you believe you can carry out your duties effectively, you should be given the opportunity to demonstrate this.
- If the amount of time you take off sick is of concern to your employer or your ability to do your job is affected, your employer may put this in writing and stop accepting sick notes, which could affect your eligibility for the company or statutory sick pay. If this happens to you, seek advice from your union or the local Citizens Advice Bureau.

How can I get advice about employment and disability rights?

The Citizens Advice Bureau is an excellent source of free advice if you feel that your employer is treating you unfairly. Solicitors specialising in employment law can also advise you but will charge, although many will give you the first half hour's advice for a fixed sum. Some may offer help and advice under the Legal Aid scheme but this does not currently cover industrial tribunal work. If you belong to a trade union, you can probably get advice from your union representative or the head office.

The Department for Work and Pensions (Social Security Agency in Northern Ireland) runs a telephone helpline that provides information on benefits for sick and disabled people and their carers. This Benefits Enquiry Line (contact details in the Appendix) can also arrange for you to ring a claimant adviser who will help you to complete the necessary forms.

Relationships

My doctor has just told me that my past smoking has caused COPD and emphysema. I don't want to be a burden – how can I tell my family and friends?

Anyone close to you is likely to experience the same initial reactions as you. However, they are probably already concerned about your health and will be relieved to know that the cause of your symptoms has been discovered.

You may want to discuss the following with them:

- COPD can be treated but not cured.
- Breathlessness is not dangerous and can be managed.
- If you do not smoke, your COPD should not get worse and you will continue more or less as normal.
- You plan to find out as much about helping yourself as possible, and take a positive approach to living with COPD.

Encourage those close to you to share their feelings with you and not to hide them. You are not the only one who will feel down; they will too.

There is help and support available to people with COPD, and to their families and carers. The British Lung Foundation is a charity that supports research into lung problems and offers help and advice to people with COPD. The patient arm of the Foundation is known as Breathe Easy. Local Breathe Easy groups organise regular meetings. These may be social events where you can meet others who face the same problems as you, and there may be an educational session with invited speakers. Many of our patients find the Breathe Easy groups a great support. Contact the British Lung Foundation to find out about your local Breathe Easy group (details in the Appendix).

My husband has severe COPD and a lot of our friends have stopped visiting. How can we show them that his breathlessness is not catching and that we need visitors?

This is a common complaint among people who have experienced any sort of chronic illness. Friends seem to be supportive if an illness is short lived, but most find it difficult to keep this up. Often they feel helpless because they can't make things better and this makes them feel uncomfortable around those who are ill. Try inviting them round for drinks or tea. This may show them that you can still enjoy a normal home life.

Think about whether you might unconsciously have excluded them in any way. It can be difficult to give time to your relationship with friends when there is illness in the family. They may think that you would actually prefer to manage on your own, especially if you always say 'we are fine'. Try to make your friends feel useful and valued, and they may come round more often!

My husband has COPD and his fear of breathlessness has started to affect our love life. I really want to help; is there anything I can do?

This must be very difficult for both of you but with your love and support your husband should be able to overcome his fear. He may well feel anxious, afraid or sad that his condition is affecting your sex life. These feelings are normal and are part of learning to live with breathlessness. An increased breathing rate during sex is normal and will not cause any harm and is not dangerous, but it is sometimes difficult to remember this. Your husband may struggle even more if he is depressed or lacking self-confidence. Although few people feel confident talking about sex, it may help to talk openly with your husband about your likes and dislikes in your love life and that you are willing to explore new and satisfying methods of fulfilment. Some people find it hard to deal with concerns about relationships but Relate (former Marriage

Guidance) can offer further advice and support. You can find the number of their nearest branch in the telephone directory.

Some possible solutions include the following.

- Plan sex when your husband's breathing is good.
- Get him to try using his 'reliever' inhaler 20 minutes before sex.
- Avoid sex when your husband is tired.
- Do not rush.
- Try different positions to reduce effort.
- Use relaxation techniques (e.g. massage) to reduce anxiety.
- Breathing exercises can help to control your husband's breathing (see Chapter 8, *Exercise and fitness*).
- Try hugging, stroking and caressing as a means of expressing yourselves.
- If your husband is very short of breath, get him to see his doctor in case his medication needs changing.
- Don't be afraid to ask for referral to someone trained to help with sexual problems.

Coping with incontinence

Sometimes my cough is so bad that I wet myself. It's very embarrassing.

We bet it is. This is particularly a problem experienced by women, especially those who have had children. When you cough, pressures inside your chest and abdomen increase very suddenly. If your bladder or pelvic muscles are weakened in any way, you can quite easily wet yourself. Although it can be embarrassing, it's not usually a sign of any medical problem affecting your pelvis, rather a sign that your COPD is not well controlled and that you require more treatment. We know that this 'stress incontinence' can be difficult to discuss with your doctor or nurse, but it is a relatively common problem so they are likely to be sympathetic and will probably review your treatment. A practical tip that some people have found useful is to try to make sure you go to the toilet regularly throughout the day, so that your bladder is never full!

Complementary therapies

Might complementary medicine have anything to offer me and my COPD?

In recent years, some forms of complementary therapy have become widely accepted by conventional medical practitioners. Therapies such as acupuncture and homoeopathy are now available in some NHS hospitals and health centres. In fact, the holistic approach of the complementary therapies – treating the whole person, mind, body and spirit – is something to which most conventional doctors and nurses aspire, even within the limited time available for each patient.

Any therapy that makes you feel better without serious side-effects can only be a good thing. The effects, good and bad, of some therapies such as Chinese medicine and herbalism are unknown because they have not undergone the stringent testing required of conventional medicines. All therapies should, however, be complementary – in addition to, and not an alternative to, your prescribed treatment.

No complementary therapy can cure COPD, but some are beneficial in improving quality of life and well-being. Symptoms such as anxiety, tension, poor sleep, lack of energy and tension headaches can often be improved by complementary therapies. The hospice movement has embraced therapies such as aromatherapy for these reasons. The important thing is to use these treatments carefully and wisely, and to make sure that the person giving them is fully trained.

My daughter paid for me to have an aromatherapy massage for my birthday. It made me feel very relaxed. Is aromatherapy suitable for people with COPD?

Any treatment that makes you feel relaxed and increases your sense of well-being is certainly good for you. Massage helps the circulation and can relieve stress and tension in your muscles. As breathlessness increases muscle tension and workload, this therapy may be especially beneficial. The aromatic plant oils used in aromatherapy can affect your emotions, encouraging pleasant thoughts and sensations, and thus increasing the benefit of massage.

My friend is interested in homoeopathy. What is it, and could it help my COPD?

Homoeopathy is a therapeutic system that has been in use for over 200 years. It works on the principle of 'like treats like'. In other words, an illness is treated with a medicine that could produce similar symptoms in a healthy person. Although this sounds a little scary, there are modern conventional drugs that work exactly on this principle. Digitalis (Digoxin), for example, can cure or cause heart irregularities.

The active ingredients are given in a highly diluted form to prevent toxicity and homoeopathic remedies are virtually 100 per cent safe. Homoeopathy is successful in treating a wide range of conditions.

Homoeopathic doctors use history taking, examination and investigation, just as all doctors do. Prescribing is then based on a wide range of aspects of the patient's condition, including the patient's personality, physical features, the effects of a variety of environmental influences, and lifestyle and social relationships.

Homoeopathy integrates well with conventional medicine and should be viewed as complementary, not alternative, treatment. There is little research evidence to show specific benefits of homoeopathic remedies on people with COPD, but it should not be detrimental to your condition as long as you do not stop taking your conventional medication. To find a qualified homoeopath contact the British Homeopathic Association (contact details in the Appendix).

10
Getting help

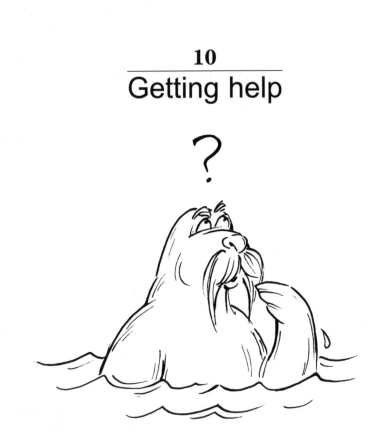

It may be that you qualify for some sort of help – financial or otherwise – from the state benefits system or from other organisations. Finding out what is available, what you are eligible for and applying for this help can be complicated. People who might be able to help you through the benefits maze are the Citizens Advice Bureau, a welfare rights worker or a social worker. Your GP surgery may have somebody helpful as part of their primary health-care team.

The Department for Work and Pensions (DWP) has helpful leaflets and booklets, including a general introductory guide.

These are available from your nearest DWP office or JobCentre. If you have access to the Internet, or have a friend or relative who has, look up their website (address in the Appendix). They have tried to make the information easy to understand, and you can even download the application forms straight onto your computer.

Because the benefits system is a complex subject, we cannot cover every aspect but we have tried to summarise the benefits that are most likely to be helpful to people with COPD and their family and carers. Our list of benefits is not exhaustive or detailed, so please regard the information that follows as general advice, and use relevant pamphlets, welfare benefit advisers, websites or helplines to check the 'small print'.

Dad has severe COPD and Mum is quite elderly. They want to stay in their own home but are finding things difficult. How much special equipment for disabled people is available on the NHS, and how much will they have to pay for it?

A certain amount of equipment for people having difficulties with their daily activities is available free of charge from the NHS or from occupational therapy services provided by the local authority social services department. Such equipment is usually provided on an open-ended loan basis: when it is no longer needed, it is returned. Items included in this sort of provision are some types of seating and aids for bathing. Sloping ramps for wheelchair access to a property or rails and handles to help with stairs and doorways may also be included.

More expensive items or ones that would require adaptations to the property are likely to involve your parents being assessed financially to see if they are able to contribute to the cost; for example, fitting a shower cubicle. In some cases your parents might be assessed as being able to afford the full cost and would be expected to pay it themselves.

I really don't want to go into residential care and would much prefer to stay at home. But my savings are very limited and I do need some new furniture to help me stay independent – my old bed is awful. Is there any financial help I can get?

If you're receiving Income Support or Jobseekers Allowance you may be able to claim a Community Care grant. This is to help with needs such as clothing and things for your home.

People who need to move home because of their disability, who wish to stay at home rather than go into residential accommodation or whose family is under exceptional pressure due to family break-down or long-term illness may be entitled to these grants. These are means-tested and if you have savings of more than £500 (more than £1,000 if you're over 60) the amount you may receive is affected.

For information and claim forms, contact your local office of the Department for Work and Pensions or see their website (see the Appendix)

Help with medical needs

I'm still working and find that my prescription charges are quite expensive now that I'm on extra inhalers. What is the cheapest way to get my medicines?

Count how many prescription items you have to get in a year. At present the prescription charge is £6.40 per item. If you pay for at least 15 prescription items a year (which would cost you a total of £96), you would be better off buying a pre-payment certificate – often called a 'season ticket' – which is £91.80 for a year or £33.40 for four months). You can get the necessary application form (form FP95) from main post offices, your primary care trust (PCT) headquarters, most chemists/pharmacist shops or, if you have access to the Internet, try the Department of Health website (address in the Appendix).

But do first check whether you are entitled to Working Tax Credit (see the next answer). This benefit can be claimed when you are working and entitles you to free prescriptions.

My neighbour gets her medicines free because she is diabetic. Is there any chance that I'm entitled to free prescriptions too?

The people who are entitled to free prescriptions are:

- over 60, or under 16, or under 19 and in full-time education; or under 25 if you live in Wales;
- pregnant, or have given birth within the last year;
- have certain medical conditions that qualify for an exemption certificate; these include diabetes, epilepsy and certain hormone deficiencies;
- a war disablement pensioner needing treatment for the war disablement;
- on a low income (apply on form HC1);
- receiving Working Tax Credit (combines what was Working Families Tax Credit and Disabled Persons Tax Credit);
- the partner of someone receiving Income Support or Jobseekers Allowance.

I don't qualify for free prescriptions and the prescription charge seems quite a lot of money to pay for everything I need.

It's natural to feel a bit aggrieved at having to pay for medicines but things could be worse if you had to pay their full cost! Below are some typical basic drug costs (correct at time of writing):

- Combivent inhaler £6.45
- Combivent nebuliser solution £31.35 for 60 vials
- Becotide 200 inhaler £19.61
- Symbicort 400 inhaler £38
- Seretide 500 inhaler £44.00
- Serevent 25 inhaler £28.60

So you can see that you get pretty good value from the NHS prescription charge, which is the same, however expensive your medication is.

I heard the practice nurse at the GP surgery talking about Health Benefits. What are they?

'Health Benefits' is a term used to describe a group of useful state benefits that go together. They include:

- free prescriptions,
- help with costs of dental treatment and eye tests,
- help towards the cost of glasses or contact lenses,
- help with costs of hospital travel (e.g. for outpatient treatment),
- help with NHS wigs.

You automatically qualify for this group of benefits if you receive Jobseekers Allowance, Income Support or New Tax Credit. You can also claim if you are in need and outside these groups. Certificate HC2 confirms that you are entitled to these benefits – you get it from your local office of the Department for Work and Pensions (DWP).

Can I still claim Health Benefits even if I have some savings?

Health Benefits are not payable if you have capital (savings and investments) over £8,000 (£12,000 if you are over 60) and live at home. This limit is increased to £18,500 for people in residential care.

Help with work

How do you go off sick? I've never taken any sick leave before but am now finding my full-time job too much for me.

If you need less than a week off work, you simply submit a 'self-certificate', which is available at your place of work. Occasionally, employers may insist on a medical certificate for periods less than a week; these are usually unnecessary and your GP is entitled to charge you for a 'private' note of this kind.

For longer than a full working week, see your GP. He or she can give you a sick certificate (commonly known as a Med 3). This may be a 'closed' sick note stating that you will be able to return to work within the next 14 days, or an 'open' sick note, which can be for longer periods.

If you have a Statutory Sick Pay (SSP) scheme at work, this sick note entitles you to receive SSP. Otherwise it entitles you to Incapacity Benefit (sickness benefit) for the period of your illness.

You mentioned that full-time working is proving too much for you. Your personnel department or, if available, your occupational health department will be able to advise you about adjusting your working hours, whether it is possible to work part-time, and about the pros and cons of early retirement.

Can my doctor give me a backdated sick note? I'm recovering from an exacerbation, and there seems to be a gap in my certificates from when I came out of hospital.

In these circumstances your GP can give you a backdated sick-note (which is known in the trade as a Med 5). Your GP must give today's date on the form but is able to state that you were ill before this.

What is a Med 4? The social security people have asked me to get one from my GP.

You may be asked to provide one of these if you are off sick for a longer period of, say, a few months. This gives your GP the opportunity to pass on more medical information than the initial certificate (Med 3) and helps the Department for Work and Pensions in deciding whether they need to review your case in person.

What is Statutory Sick Pay?

Unless they are in an Occupational Sick Pay scheme, most people in employment will receive Statutory Sick Pay for six months (28 weeks) from their employer when they are off sick. The amount of Statutory Sick Pay is set by government and is not related to what you are earning. People who do not have an employer – for example, the self-employed or those who are out of work – are not eligible for SSP but can claim state Incapacity Benefit instead.

What happens if I am off sick for longer than 28 weeks?

Once 28 weeks of sickness have elapsed, you receive Incapacity Benefit instead of SSP. Income Support (which is means-tested) may also be payable if you're off sick.

How do they tell whether I qualify for Incapacity Benefit and the other benefits?

During the first 28 weeks of illness or incapacity the *Own Occupation Test* is applied. This determines whether – because of your illness – you are incapable of the sort of work you would be expected to do in the course of your usual job.

After 28 weeks of sick leave (for most people) the *All Work Test* applies. This is to decide whether your illness reduces your ability to carry out a general range of work-related activities. You are sent a questionnaire (called an IB50) that asks about your level of ability and about any difficulties you would encounter in a wide variety of activities, such as walking, standing up, lifting, managing stairs, speech, hearing and continence. The questionnaire is quite long and detailed, so it may be helpful to go through it with a friend or relative.

Does my being off sick for more than 28 weeks mean I will be called up by the Department for Work and Pensions for a physical examination?

The Department for Work and Pensions (DWP) is often able to decide whether you would pass or fail the All Work Test purely with the help of the IB50 questionnaire (see the answer above) and a report from your doctor. You might be asked to request a Med 4 form from your doctor for this purpose. Only if more

information is needed would you then be asked to see a DWP
doctor for an examination. No one is refused benefit without
being offered an examination, and you have the right of appeal if
you are not happy with the result.

Who gets Income Support?

You may be eligible for Income Support if you are:

*   over 60,
*   only able to work part-time or cannot work at all because
    of a disability,
*   a single parent,
*   caring for someone who is elderly, sick or disabled,

and you have limited savings of less than £8,000.

Receiving Income Support is a gateway to other sources of help;
as well as a cash payment, it entitles you to free prescriptions,
eye tests, dental treatment, school meals, help with the cost of
spectacles, and some other benefits.

**I've been off sick from work for some time after a couple
of exacerbations and I am getting Incapacity Benefit now.
I would like to try doing some paid work, perhaps just for
a day or two a week, but I don't want to risk giving up my
benefits until I'm sure I can cope.**

If you are receiving Incapacity Benefit there are rules about
'Permitted Work'. Under these rules you are allowed to work for up
to 16 hours per week and earn a maximum of £66 a week for a limit
of six months to see whether you're ready for the world of work yet.

This period can be extended if it is likely to improve your
ability to work full-time, with permission from someone at the
Department for Work and Pensions such as a Disability
Employment Adviser. However, you can earn a maximum of £20
a week indefinitely. Permitted Work is a useful way of getting
yourself back into some work at your own pace and building up
your confidence.

**Because of my COPD, my breathlessness is much worse
and now I can only manage to work half-time. Is there
any help I can get to top up my earnings? I really don't
want to go off sick again.**

You may be eligible for Working Tax Credit, which is adminis-
tered by Inland Revenue. If you're working at least 16 hours a
week, have an illness that puts you at a disadvantage in getting a
job and have limited savings, you should consider applying for
this tax-free benefit.

You need to have been receiving certain other benefits first.
These include Incapacity Benefit, Housing Benefit, Jobseekers
Allowance and some other incapacity benefits. It is means-tested:
you cannot apply for it if you have more than £8,000 in savings,
and the amount you receive will be affected if you have more
than £3,000 in savings. There is also a 'fast track' version of this
benefit, aimed at making it financially possible for you to get
back to work on reduced earnings. To get more information
about Working Tax Credit, contact the New Tax Credit helpline
(details in the Appendix).

**My workmates have suggested I ask our Occupational
Health Department for advice and help, as I'm worried
that I'll have difficulty in getting back to work after my
last hospital stay with a severe exacerbation. What can
they do to help me?**

Many large employers have their own occupational health department (OHD). Even small firms may have an arrangement with the
local Occupational Health Department to provide this form of
help for their employees.

An occupational health doctor is someone who is independent
of both management on the one hand and the individual on the
other. They are experienced in making the workplace fit the
employee (rather than the other way round!). If someone has an
illness or disability, the OHD can look at the implications of this
and find ways of making the workplace easier. Some examples of
this include:

- starting back at work on a part-time basis after a severe illness;
- working flexitime and travelling to and from work out of the rush hour, if mobility is a problem;
- to work on the ground floor if no lift is available for someone who has difficulty with stairs.

Special chairs or pieces of equipment may be suggested, or a move to a different department may be helpful.

I'm currently off sick and have been advised that I will have to give up work because of COPD. What benefits am I entitled to?

Someone who is incapable of work because of sickness or disability, either temporarily or permanently, may qualify for one of the following state benefits:

- Statutory Sick Pay,
- Incapacity Benefit.

These benefits are intended to provide an income for a person who cannot work. Only one can be paid at any given time but you might also be able to claim an income-related benefit (such as Disability Living Allowance) as well. The rules are complex and you will need extra help and advice from your employer, the Citizens Advice Bureau or the local office of the Department for Work and Pensions (formerly called the Benefits Agency) to make sure that you are claiming correctly.

Statutory Sick Pay (SSP) is paid by an employer to an employee who is not yet 65 years of age and cannot work because of sickness or disability, and is earning at least as much as the National Insurance lower earnings limit. SSP can be paid from the first day off work for 28 weeks. If your employment ends while you are receiving SSP, you may be able to claim Incapacity Benefit instead.

Incapacity Benefit is paid to someone aged under 60 (for a woman) or 65 (for a man) who cannot work because of sickness or disability but is not entitled to SSP and has paid sufficient National Insurance contributions. There are three types of Incapacity Benefit:

- *Lower rate short-term*: paid for the first 196 days of sickness, and an additional payment can be made for an adult dependant.
- *Higher rate short-term*: paid from day 197 to day 364. Again, an additional payment can be made for an adult dependant.
- *Longer-term*: paid from day 365 of sickness. Additional payments can be made for an adult dependant, child(ren) and age.

For the first 196 days you would have to show that you were incapable of work by sending in medical certificates. After 196 days you would normally have to have a medical examination and assessment to confirm that you are unable to work.

The contribution conditions for Incapacity Benefit are complicated. If you are not sure whether you meet the conditions for entitlement, contact the Benefits Enquiry Line (details in the Appendix) or your local Citizens Advice Bureau.

Disability Living Allowance is paid to people under the age of 65 who have care or mobility needs. It is intended to help with the extra costs of disability, and is not means-tested. The claim form for this allowance is lengthy and you can get help with filling it in from the Benefits Enquiry Line (contact details in the Appendix) or consult an experienced adviser at the Citizens Advice Bureau.

Help for people at home and their carers

Although my neighbours have promised to help as much as possible, I'm worried about how I'll cope when I get home from hospital. Is there any way that I can get some help?

Ask one of the ward staff to get in touch with a social worker for
you. Some hospitals have their own social workers but in other
areas it will be a social worker in your local authority's social services department. If you cannot afford to pay for private care, it
may be possible for the local authority social services to arrange
for 'domiciliary help'. This will provide home care services such
as help with getting up, going to bed, managing housework and,
sometimes, doing the shopping. A social worker will do a 'care
management assessment' to find out what your needs are and
decide what services can be provided. Services such as visits
from the district nurse to help with dressings are free, but a
charge may be made for some non-medical care services. Be
warned, though, that funding is usually very limited and these
services can be provided only for people in the greatest need.

If social services can help you, they will draw up a care
package that outlines what will be supplied. In some instances
(usually more in situations requiring long-term care), rather than
arranging for the care direct, the local authority will give the individual the money allocated so that she or he can choose the services to be used. This would be unlikely to happen in your case,
though, as we hope that you will need help only in the relatively
short term.

Make sure that ward staff are aware of your concerns before
you are ready to leave, so that they can plan the necessary
support for you to be ready and waiting for you on your return
home.

What is the Disability Living Allowance – DLA? Would I be eligible for it?

People under the age of 65 who have a significant disability may
be able to claim this benefit. It has two parts: the Care component
and the Mobility component.

The *Care component* is for people who need a considerable
amount of help with personal care, such as dressing, preparing a
cooked meal, using the toilet or getting into or out of bed. There
are three levels of benefit: the lowest rate is for someone who
needs help during the day, the middle rate is for someone needing

help during the day or the night, and the highest is for someone who needs help both day and night.

The *Mobility component* is worth applying for if your disability has continued for longer than six months, and you cannot walk or have difficulty in walking even short distances. This could apply to someone with COPD whose breathlessness has become so severe that they cannot walk even a short distance without having to stop.

DLA is not taxed or means-tested and it can be used in any way you wish. You might choose to use it to help with the costs of taxis or to help with petrol costs if friends give you lifts. It can also be used towards the cost of running a car under the Motability scheme (discussed later, under 'Help for car users').

My mother is over 65 and so is not eligible for Disability Living Allowance. Is there any other benefit that she can get?

She should apply for Attendance Allowance (AA). She may be entitled to this if she is severely disabled and has needed a great deal of care for at least six months. To qualify for this benefit she needs frequent help, or continual supervision throughout the day to keep herself safe. Needing help with eating or drinking, washing, showering or bathing, or getting about indoors would all qualify her for this benefit.

Someone who repeatedly needs help at night – for example, help to get to the lavatory – would also qualify.

Application forms are available from the local office of the Department for Work and Pensions. Your mother might be asked to have a medical examination, which can be arranged in her own home if necessary.

A Carer's Special Grant may also be available to help you take a short break from caring for your mother.

Mum has become progressively disabled and I've had to give up my work to look after her at home. It's virtually a full-time job being her carer. She does get Attendance Allowance but she'd have to go into a nursing home if I

wasn't looking after her, and neither of us wants that. As Mum's carer, am I entitled to any benefits?

A 'carer' is anyone who looks after a relative, partner, spouse or even friend, of any age, who cannot manage without some help. The person you're looking after can be an adult or a child and it does not matter if you're over or under 65.

Anyone who cares for someone for at least 35 hours per week and is under the age of 65, with earnings of not more than £75 per week, may be eligible for Carer's Allowance. They do have to pay Income Tax on this allowance (depending, of course, on any other earnings). It is not means-tested so it does not depend on any savings they may have. The person they are caring for has to be receiving Attendance Allowance (AA) or the higher rate of Disability Living Allowance (DLA).

So, yes, you should certainly apply for Carer's Allowance.

Would the person I'm looking after have their benefit reduced if I claim Carer's Allowance?

In some circumstances – but not invariably – their benefit might be reduced if you claim this allowance. Ask for a benefit check to see whether it is worth claiming Carer's Allowance; a welfare benefits adviser should be able to help you do this. Ask at your local Department for Work and Pensions or Citizens Advice Bureau, or try the Benefits Enquiry Line or Carer's Allowance helpline (see the Appendix).

My partner and I have been looking after Dad for years and have never had a break. Is there any sort of help that can we get?

It is extremely important that you get a break from looking after your dad. Being a carer is emotionally and physically taxing, and carers have high levels of stress and depression and are more prone to infection. Day-to-day help can be provided by social services home care or private agencies. Your GP or health visitor should be able to make a referral to social services on your behalf or you could find the number in the phone book and contact them direct. Some of the voluntary organisations such as Crossroads Caring for Carers (contact details in the Appendix) provide sitting services at home and in some areas occasional overnight care so you can get some time to yourself, and a good night's sleep too if your dad needs you at night.

It is also sensible to have some longer breaks on a regular basis. This is called respite care and would involve your dad going to stay in a care home for a week or two at a time. This could be organised by your GP, health visitor or social worker.

I had to retire early because of my COPD. I was the main breadwinner and so it's been hard to keep our family home together. We've had a bad roof leak, and the insurance company won't pay for all the damage. What on earth can we do?

You may be able to apply to the Department for Work and Pensions for a Crisis Loan from the Social Fund. It is aimed at giving you help in an emergency or disaster, which would otherwise affect the health and safety of you or your family. You do not need to be receiving any other benefits to get this. Although you do have to pay the loan back over time, it is interest-free.

Help for car users

How can I get a disabled parking bay for Mum? She has great difficulty in walking and the parking around here is terrible.

If your mum has no reasonable off-street parking, bays or lines can be installed outside her home if:

- she has a Blue (or Orange) parking badge and lives where the parking space is required;
- she can prove regular and frequent use of the vehicle, either by herself or by her carer as driver (you, perhaps?), who must live at the same address.

The Blue (formerly Orange) Badge parking scheme is run by the local authority. It also entitles your mum to park safely for a limited time where parking is otherwise prohibited (e.g. on double yellow lines) so that she can shop. She needs to have significant difficulty with mobility to be eligible for this scheme.

An application form is available from her local authority offices, or ask at her nearest post office, Department for Work and Pensions or social services department. Remember that she can use this badge if somebody gives her a lift: she is entitled to put it in someone else's car as long as she is using it at the time. This can make her a welcome passenger!

I've heard about something called the Motability scheme, for people who have difficulty in getting around. How can I find out more about this to help me?

If you receive the higher rate Mobility component of the Disability Living Allowance, you can use this benefit to take part in the Motability scheme. Car manufacturers, motor insurers and providers of finance take part in this scheme, which is aimed at helping people with a disability obtain a suitable vehicle for their needs.

Contract hire and hire purchase schemes are available for new and used vehicles, and Motability also helps with hire purchase for powered wheelchairs and scooters. By handing over part or all of your benefit you can be provided with a vehicle to suit your needs.

Depending on your financial circumstances, charitable grants may also be available to help with the cost of acquiring a suitable vehicle, of carrying out any necessary modifications to it (such as hand controls, wheelchair access or special driver's seats), and if necessary for special driving lessons. If you cannot drive yourself but need transport, you can apply for a vehicle for your carer under this scheme.

For more information, or for details of your nearest dealer, contact Motability (details in the Appendix).

Dad is now convalescing after a very severe exacerbation of COPD – he was in intensive care for a week and in hospital for nearly three weeks in all. He is determined not to give up driving his car, and it's important for his independence. Will he be safe?

After a major illness of this sort, people do need a period of convalescence to get back on their feet and back to their usual level of activity. In general, someone recovering from illness is safe to drive once they can safely put on the brakes and control the car in an emergency – for example, if a child were to run out into the road.

Older drivers need to remember that their general level of fitness and, in particular, their eyesight must be good enough to control a car safely in today's hectic traffic. Your dad's eyesight has to be good enough for him to be able to read a number plate at 20.5 metres (25 yards). This is something that he can check quite easily for himself. If there is any doubt, he should ask for a full eye test at an optometrist's. His GP is also a good person to ask if there are any general health queries about his fitness to drive.

Dad is elderly and quite frail. How can we be sure that he is safe to drive?

COPD or physical frailty or old age does not prevent anyone from driving. However, the severity of COPD together with other health problems and the effects of ageing might raise the question of whether someone is fit to drive.

Using a car can be a lifeline for older people. But our reaction times, concentration, memory and eyesight do become less sharp as we get older. Older drivers are usually able to remain safe by recognising ageing changes of this sort in themselves and making sensible allowances, such as avoiding hectic traffic, unfamiliar routes and conditions of poor visibility.

Regular eye checks are sensible for older drivers. Someone who could not read a standard car number plate in a good light (with glasses if worn) at 20.5 metres (25 yards) would not be considered able to hold a licence. After reaching the age of 70, people must reapply for a driving licence every three years, and the

application form includes a medical questionnaire to be filled in
by the individual.

A local driving school or a disabled drivers' assessment centre
can give advice and arrange a suitable test if you are in doubt.
Your father might like to consider whether he is supporting the
expense of a car for very little use. Looking at the total annual
cost and comparing this with taxi fares over a year could be a
helpful exercise.

Do I have to notify the DVLA that I have COPD?

No, you don't. You must notify the Driver and Vehicle Licensing
Agency (DVLA) only if you have any medical condition 'that is
likely to render you a source of danger while driving'. Some specific medical conditions, such as epilepsy, are legal bars to individuals holding a licence unless certain conditions are met.

COPD on its own does not come into this category. But it is a
driver's duty to notify the DVLA of any medical condition that
might affect safe driving, so if, for example, you have severe
breathlessness with an exacerbation, you might well be unfit to
drive until you had made a good recovery.

Ask yourself whether you could safely control your car in an
emergency, such as if a child ran out into the road in front of you.
If you are in any doubt about this – for example, if you have other
medical conditions such as heart or eye problems – get advice
from your GP.

The DVLA publishes helpful information about safety to drive
and can supply you with a list of disabled driver assessment
centres. (Contact details are in the Appendix.)

Help with care homes

What happens if I have to go into a nursing home? How can I pay for this?

If someone cannot manage at home they may consider going into a
residential or nursing home – now officially called 'care home' and

'care home (nursing)'. If you feel the time is coming when you might need to consider living in a care home, talk to your local social services department. They will look at all the options, including whether it may be possible to provide extra help and support so that you can stay in your own home, at least for a bit longer.

The social services department can help you decide whether you need just residential care or regular nursing care. They can also help you choose the right sort of home, help you work out the finances and see whether you are entitled to any state benefits. If you have savings of more than £16,000 (2004 figure), you will be expected to pay the full cost (until your savings fall below that amount).

The social services department will arrange to pay the home's fees if you cannot afford to pay them yourself. But remember that some care homes' fees are higher than the level of payments available from social services. In this case, you would need to make up the difference yourself or find a home with fees that the social services are prepared to pay.

If you needed nursing care in a home, your place (or at least the nursing/medical care) might be funded by the NHS. However, this aspect of funding is a very grey area, so you will need to get advice about it. Age Concern (contact details in the Appendix) publishes information about finding and paying for care homes, which you might find useful.

Help other than state benefits

What other sources of help are there apart from the Department for Work and Pensions?

There are a surprising number of sources of help in the UK apart from the state sector. Whether you're concerned about a relative or about your own situation, you could ask the local Citizens Advice Bureau for advice. If you have checked that you are receiving all the state benefits to which you are entitled (and these benefits are often under-claimed), you may find that one of the charities will be able to help, perhaps with a one-off grant.

The book *Charities Digest* (ask for it in your local library) gives information about local and national sources of help. Were you in the armed forces? If so, SSAFA Forces Help or the Royal British Legion (see the Appendix for contact details) might be able to help. A social worker can probably guide you in the right direction. There is also a helpful document called *A Guide to Grants for Individuals in Need,* obtainable from your local office of the Department for Work and Pensions.

11
Research and the future

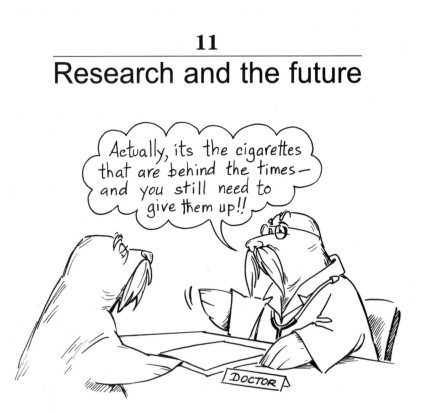

A lot of progress has been made in the treatment of COPD over the last 20 years and it is almost certain that new medicines will become available in the future. This is because we are learning more about why people get COPD and what causes the damage. All this means that there is the potential to develop new and better treatments.

We are also finding that drugs currently used in the treatment of other lung diseases may also be helpful in COPD.

New treatments and methods

With all this research and development, will there be any new treatments for me?

A few specific areas deserve a special mention.

ANTIOXIDANTS

Part of the damage caused by cigarettes comes from molecules called *oxygen radicals*. These damage the air sacs and the surrounding small airways. Some recent work suggests that anti-oxidants may neutralise this process and reduce or delay the damage. Antioxidants are most easily found in diets containing lots of fruit and vegetables. They are also available in tablet form but we suspect that a good diet is probably the most efficient treatment.

PHOSPHODIESTERASE-4 (PDE4) INHIBITORS

You might have taken 'relatives' of these compounds as part of your COPD treatment. They come from the same group as aminophylline and theophylline drugs. The major problem with those products in the past has been that many people have suffered side-effects from the medication. It is hoped that these more 'refined' products will produce benefits without the side-effects.

VITAMINS

Whilst some scientists have suggested that vitamins C and E may be helpful for people with COPD, there is not enough evidence to recommend their regular use. Indeed, there has been some concern that too many vitamins can be harmful. The 'take home' message is really that we should all eat a healthy balanced diet, full of fresh fruit and vegetables!

I can't really see why I have to attend the hospital clinics. Surely my GP could give me some of the care I get in out-patients?

It's difficult to give an answer to this that reflects everybody's experiences but it is certainly true that an increasing amount of care for many chronic diseases is happening at the GP surgery and not in the hospital out-patient clinic. Some chronic diseases have had a plan formulated for them by the Department of Health. These are called National Service Frameworks (NSFs). The idea is that every surgery and hospital should supply the same quality of treatment, so that where you live will no longer affect the treatment you receive. NSFs currently exist for cancers, heart disease, diabetes and care of the elderly, but unfortunately not yet for chest diseases. We sincerely hope that this will change. In the meantime, many interested health professionals are trying to set up local systems of care for patients with COPD; most of these are centred on the general practice or health centre, with support from the local hospital.

I've got severe disease and find it very difficult to get to the hospital. Can't people come and see me at home?

Yes! There are many examples of exactly this type of care being developed up and down the country. The exciting thing is that all the various groups involved in health care and support are beginning to talk to each other in an effort to come up with a formula that everyone can use. We see no reason why the future should not see an increasing number of people with COPD being looked after outside the hospital.

It is not easy to get to the hospital where I go for spirometry. Is there any hope that this will be done at my health centre in future?

You will know from Chapter 3 (*How is COPD diagnosed?*) how important spirometry is in diagnosing COPD. Until recently there have been concerns that spirometry performed outside a hospital might not be of high enough quality to diagnose COPD.

Things are changing fast, though, and a large number of special-
ist nurses and GPs are able to use spirometry in their surgeries.
We hope that this practice will increase as the organisation of
COPD services improves as a whole.

Can anybody be screened for COPD?

For those of you who don't know about this sort of thing, the
term 'screening' means trying to find out whether people have a
particular disease, such as COPD, when they don't realise it. An
example would be to perform spirometry in everybody over the
age of 40 who smokes. This might be possible in some parts of the
UK but it is not widely available. If you are concerned that you
(or a friend or relative) might have COPD, read Chapter 1 (*What
is COPD?*) and then make an appointment with your (or their)
GP or practice nurse to discuss it.

When will they make safe cigarettes?

We suspect that the answer to that will be 'never'. Currently, your
average cigarette contains over 2,000 harmful products and is
extremely addictive. The best treatment is still going to be 'no
cigarettes'.

Surgery

Aren't there any operations for people like me?

A small number of people with COPD develop large, cyst-type
structures in the lungs, called *bullae*. Some of these can grow
large enough to interfere with nearby areas of lung and stop them
working so well. In some instances it is possible to remove these
bullae but you will require specialist review, and sometimes the
potential gains from the operation are outweighed by the risks of
the surgery and anaesthetics required.

A relatively new operation has been tried on people who have
emphysema. It is called *lung volume reduction surgery* (LVRS).

In emphysema there are lots of air spaces in the lungs that are useless in the breathing process and sometimes their removal allows other areas of lung to work more efficiently. The operation was developed in the USA and initial results have been promising. The problems at present are twofold: first, the effects do not seem to last for more than a few years; and secondly, there is no real agreement about which people should be put forward for this kind of surgery. Trials are being undertaken in the UK to answer these questions. Watch this space!

What I really need, though, is a new set of lungs. Could I have a transplant?

The issues surrounding lung transplantation are varied and complicated but we'll do our best to answer you! In theory, people with emphysema can be put forward for lung transplantation, and currently most success has been achieved by transplanting just one lung, the *single lung transplant*. The problems with this and other forms of lung transplantation are associated with the lack of donors and finding a compatible lung. Whilst the operation itself is reasonably straightforward there are lots of potential complications, with rejection of the new lung and side-effects from the drugs used after the operation. Currently, usually only people under the age of 50 with severe emphysema are put forward for consideration for transplant surgery. And they will certainly have to have stopped smoking!

Other possibilities

What is an expert patient? Can I become one?

'Expert patients' are people living with a long-term (chronic) illness, who are able to take more control over their health by understanding and managing their conditions, leading to an improved quality of life. The Expert Patient Programme was set up by the Department of Health to encourage people with chronic diseases, such as COPD, to feel more confident about their condition and to enter more into a partnership with their doctor or other health-care workers in its management. Expert Patient courses take place over 2½ hours per week for six weeks and are led by people who, themselves, live with a long-term health condition.

If you are interested in this, get in touch with the Expert Patient Programme direct (contact details in the Appendix).

Research studies

Can I be a guinea-pig to help other people?

Many hospitals and GP surgeries are involved in research aiming to find out more about the causes of, and the treatments for, COPD. Some of this research involves carrying out surveys to see how people cope and others involve tests to find out why someone has COPD when someone else does not; others certainly involve research into potential new drug treatments.

Your doctor is likely to know someone to contact if you are interested, and sometimes advertisements are placed in the newspapers, asking for 'volunteers'. A word of caution, though. Make sure that the establishment you go to has proper procedures in place. Each and every study should be clearly explained and you should be given written information and time to ask questions. If you are happy to take part, you will be asked to sign a consent form, a copy of which is for you to keep. You should also be seen by the 'lead' doctor or a member of the team to check whether you have any queries. This type of research is often called a 'clinical trial' and is a very important part of our quest to improve treatments for COPD.

Glossary

Words in *italic* in the definitions are also defined in this Glossary.

acute In a medical context, this means short term (see also *chronic*)

aerobic Requiring oxygen

alpha-1 antitrypsin A protein (produced by the liver) that enters the bloodstream – its main role is to protect the lungs from damage by other proteins called enzymes; when alpha-1 antitrypsin is deficient, the lung is poorly protected from the enzymes and loss of lung tissue occurs, leading to emphysema

alveoli Tiny air sacs in the lungs

anticholinergics Drugs that decrease the amount of mucus and phlegm you make, which often makes you feel better; they also help the muscles in the airways to relax, making the airways wider and thus helping your breathing

antioxidants Substances that are thought to help the body to 'mop up' harmful things we breathe in (or eat) and prevent damage occurring to our healthy cells

beta-agonists Drugs that cause the muscles in the airways to relax, which can make the airways wider and thus help breathing

bronchial hyper-reactivity A tendency of the smooth muscle of the trachea and bronchi to contract more intensely to a given stimulus than it does in normal individuals

bronchiectasis A *chronic* lung condition characterised by the production of large amounts of phlegm, often as a result of a previous serious infection

bronchodilator A drug that opens up the airways

bullae Large, cyst-type structures in the lungs

capillaries The smallest blood vessels

chronic In a medical context, this means long term (see also *acute*)

cilia Little hair-like structures that beat away irritants from the airways

cor pulmonale The medical term for severe COPD causing low oxygen and changes to the performance of your heart

course Refers to the medication you are prescribed to take for a certain period of time; e.g. 'a course of steroids' might be taking 6 or 8 steroid tablets a day for two weeks

emphysema A lung condition in which large numbers of the *alveoli* have been destroyed, resulting in much less area for *gas exchange* to take place

gas exchange The exchange of oxygen for carbon dioxide in the *alveoli* of the lungs

hypoxaemia Another name for 'hypoxia', which see

hypoxia A low level of oxygen in the blood

passive smoking Breathing in somebody else's cigarette smoke

pleura The lining of the lungs

primary care trust The local organisation that works with agencies that provide health care – GPs, community nurses, health visitors, dentists, optometrists and pharmacists – to ensure that the community's health needs are met.

Appendix
Useful addresses

Only some of the organisations listed below have been mentioned in the text. They are included here, however, in case you might find them useful. Please note that addresses, especially website addresses, change from time to time.

Age Concern England
1268 London Road
London SW16 4ER
Information line: 0800 00 99 66
Tel: 020 8765 7200
Fax: 020 8765 7211
Website:
www.ageconcern.org.uk
Provides advice and support on a range of subjects for people over 50

Assist UK (formerly **Disabled Living Centres Council**)
Redbank House
4 St Chad's Street
Cheetham
Manchester M8 8QA
Tel: 0870 770 2866
Textphone: 0870 770 5813
Fax: 0870 770 2867
Website: www.dlcc.org.uk
Co-ordinates the work of Disabled Living Centres UK-wide, which have information and advice about products that can increase disabled or older people's choices about how they live. Offers training courses for professionals.

Bandolier
Website: www.ebandolier.com
An e-journal with the latest
evidence-based research data
on a wide variety of subjects.
Written for doctors so it is
quite technical, but very
readable for anyone who is
interested in science.

Benefits Enquiry Line
(BEL)
Helpline: 0800 88 22 00
  N. Ireland: 0800 220 674
Textphone: 0800 243 355
Website: www.dwp.gov.uk
Government agency giving
information and advice on
sickness and disability
benefits for people with
disabilities and their carers.

Breathe Easy Club
British Lung Foundation
73–75 Goswell Road
London EC1V 7ER
Tel: 020 7688 5555
Fax: 020 7688 5556
Website: www.lunguk.org
Self-help groups for social
contact, support and
encouragement

British Homeopathic
Association
Hahneman House
29 Park Street West
Luton LU1 3BE
Tel: 0870 444 3950
Fax: 0870 444 3960
Website:
www.trusthomeopathy.org
Professional body offering
lists of qualified
homoeopathic practitioners.

British Hypnotherapy
Association
67 Upper Berkeley Street
London W1H 7QX
Tel: 020 7723 4443
Website: www.british-
hypnotherapy-association.org
Professional body of
registered hypnotherapists
who have undergone at least
four years' training in
hypnotherapy. Offers full
information about
hypnotherapy and how it
could help.

British Legion
see Royal British Legion

British Lung Foundation
73–75 Goswell Road
London EC1V 7ER
Helpline: 08458 50 50 20
Tel: 020 7688 5555
Fax: 020 7688 5556
Website: www.lunguk.org
*Association of professionals
who fund medical research
and provide support and
information to people with
lung disease. Offers leaflets
about suitable gentle
exercises and breathing
control.*

**British Medical
Acupuncture Society**
BMAS House
3 Winnington Court
Northwich
Cheshire CW8 1AQ
Tel: 01606 786782
Fax: 01606 786783
Website: www.medical-
acupuncture.co.uk
*Professional body offering
training to doctors, and list
of accredited acupuncture
practitioners.*

CareDirect
Freephone: 0800 444000
Website:
www.caredirect.gov.uk
*Operates only in southwest
England. A one-stop phone
service for people over 60,
giving information and
advice about benefits and
pensions, how to get help at
home and general health
advice. Can put you in touch
with other relevant
organisations.*

Carers Allowance
Department for Work and
Pensions
Palatine House
Lancaster Road
Preston PR1 1HB
Helpline: 01253 856123
Website: www.dwp.gsi.gov.uk
*Government helpline giving
information about Carer's
Allowance (formerly the
Invalid Care Allowance).*

Carers UK
20–25 Glasshouse Yard
London EC1A 4JT
Helpline: 0808 808 7777
(10–12 a.m., 2–4 p.m., Wed &
Thurs only)
Tel: 020 7490 8818
Fax: 020 7490 8824
Website:
www.carersonline.org.uk
Information and support for
all people who are unpaid
carers: those looking after
others with medical or other
problems. Campaigns at
national level on behalf of all
carers.
The Association has various
regional centres as follows:

CARERS NORTH OF ENGLAND
23 New Mount Street
Manchester M4 4DE
Tel: 0161 953 4233
Fax: 0161 953 4092
Website:
www.carersonline.org.uk

CARERS NORTHERN IRELAND
58 Howard Street
Belfast BT1 6PJ
Tel: 028 9043 9843
Fax: 028 9043 9299
Website:
www.carersonline.org.uk

CARERS SCOTLAND
91 Mitchell Street
Glasgow G1 3LN
Helpline: 0808 808 7777
Tel: 0141 221 9141
Fax: 0141 221 9140
Website:
www.carersonline.org.uk

CARERS WALES
River House
Ynysbridge Court
Gwaelod y Garth
Cardiff CF15 9SS
Tel: 029 2081 1370
Fax: 029 2081 1575
Website:
www.carersonline.org.uk

Chest, Heart and Stroke
Association (Northern
Ireland)
21 Dublin Road
Belfast BT2 7HB
Helpline: 0845 769 7297
Fax: 028 9033 3487
Website: www.nichsa.com
For information and advice.

Chest, Heart and Stroke
Association (Scotland)
65 North Castle Street
Edinburgh EH2 3LT
AdviceLine: 0845 077 6000
Fax: 0131 220 6313
Website: www.chss.org.uk
For information and advice.

Citizens Advice (National Association – NACAB)
Myddleton House
115–123 Pentonville Road
London N1 9LZ
Tel: 020 7833 2181
Fax: 020 7833 4371
Website:
www.adviceguide.org.uk
Headquarters of the Citizens Advice Bureaux. Has network of local branches throughout the UK, which offer a wide variety of practical, financial and legal advice. Listed in phone books and in Yellow Pages *under 'Counselling and advice'.*

Complementary Medical Association
67 Eagle Heights
The Falcons
Bramlands Close
London SW11 2LJ
Helpline: 0845 129 8434
Tel: 0845 129 8435
Website: www.the-cma.org.uk
A not-for-profit medical body offering membership to highly qualified practitioners of complementary medicine. Has a database of accredited practitioners around the UK.

Crossroads Caring for Carers
10 Regent Place
Rugby
Warwickshire CV21 2PN
Helpline: 0845 450 0350
Tel: 01788 573 653
  Wales 02920 222 282
Fax: 01788 565 498
Website:
www.crossroads.org.uk
Supports and delivers services for carers and people with care needs, via its local branches.

Crossroads (Scotland) Care Attendance Schemes
24 George Square
Glasgow G2 1EG
Tel: 0141 226 3793
Fax: 0141 221 7130
Website:
www.crossroads.scotland.co.uk
Offers information and practical support to carers and people with care needs in Scotland.

Department of Health
Richmond House
79 Whitehall
London SW1A 2NS
Helpline: 0800 555 777
Tel: 020 7210 4850
Textphone: 020 7210 5025
Fax: 01623 724 524
Website: www.doh.gov.uk
*Produces literature about
health issues, available via
the helpline. Also*
www.doh.gov.uk/nhscharges
*for information about
prescription charges and
prepayment certificates,
including the application
form FP95.
To apply for the European
Health Insurance Card, see
the website or ring 0845 606
2030. They need your name,
date of birth and NHS or
National Insurance number.*

Department for Transport
Disability Policy Branch,
Mobility and Inclusion Unit
Zone 1/18 Great Minster
House
76 Marsham Street
London SW1P 4DR
Tel: 020 7944 2914
Helpdesk: 020 7944 8300
Fax: 020 7944 9643
Website: www.mobility-
unit.dft.gov.uk

*Recorded message refers to
social services at local
councils for information
about the Blue Badge parking
scheme.*

**Department for Work and
Pensions**
Richmond House
79 Whitehall
London SW1A 2NS
Tel: 020 7210 4850
Textphone: 020 7210 5025
Fax: 01623 724 524
Benefits Enquiry Line: 0800 88
22 00
Website: www.dwp.gov.uk
*Government department
giving information about,
and claim forms for, all state
benefits.*

Disability Living Allowance
Department for Work and
Pensions
Palatine House
Lancaster Road
Preston PR1 1HB
Helpline: 08457 123 456
Tel: 020 7712 2171
Fax: 020 7712 2386
Website: www.dwp.gov.uk
*Government department
giving advice about
Disability Living Allowance.*

Disability Rights Commission
FREEPOST
MID 02164
Stratford upon Avon CV37 9BR
Tel: 08457 622633
Textphone: 08457 622 644 (8 a.m.–8 p.m., weekdays
Fax: 08457 778878
Website: www.drc-gb.org
Government-sponsored centre with publications and information on the Disability Discrimination Act. A special team of advisers can help with problems of discrimination at work.

Disability Living Centres Council *see* Assist UK

Disabled Living Foundation
380–384 Harrow Road
London W9 2HU
Helpline: 0845 130 9177 (10 a.m.–1 p.m., weekdays)
Tel: 020 7289 6111
Fax: 020 7266 2922
Textphone: 020 7432 8009
Website: www.dlf.org.uk
Information for disabled and older people on all kinds of equipment that will promote their independence and quality of life.

DVLA (Driver and Vehicle Licensing Agency)
Medical Branch
Longview Road
Morriston
Swansea SA99 1TU
Helpline: 0870 600 0301
Tel: 0870 240 0009
Fax: 01792 761100
Website: www.dvla.gov.uk
Government office offering advice to drivers with medical conditions.

Expert Patient Programme
Tel: 0845 606 6040
Website: www.expertpatients.nhs.uk
Department of Health project that helps people with a long-term condition to feel more confident about it and to enter more into a partnership with their doctor and other health-care workers in its management. Can refer people to courses around the country addressing the consequences of living with long-term illnesses.

Extend
2 Place Farm
Wheathampstead
Herts AL4 8SB
Tel/Fax: 01582 832760
Website: www.extend.org.uk
*Promotes exercise to music
for older people, and for
disabled people of all ages.
Offers video package for
people who are housebound
and cannot attend local
classes. Also arranges
training courses.*

Foundations
Bleaklow House
Howard Town Mill
Glossop SK13 8HT
Tel: 01457 891909
Fax: 01457 869361
Website:
www.foundations.uk.com
*Co-ordinates home
improvement agencies
throughout England. Can
refer older or disabled home
owners and private-sector
tenants on low incomes to
local authorities for free
repairs or improvements to
premises to enable them to
stay in their own homes.*

Health Development Agency
71 High Holborn
London WC1V 6NA
Helpline: 0870 121 4194
Tel: 020 7067 5800
Fax: 020 7061 3390
Website: www.hda-
online.org.uk
*Formerly the Health
Education Authority; it now
deals only with research.
Publications on health
matters can be ordered on
0800 555 777.*

Keep Fit Association (KFA)
Astra House Suite 1.05
Arklow Road
London SE14 6EB
Tel: 020 8692 9566
Fax: 020 8692 8383
Website: www.keepfit.org.uk
*Offers information and
training courses to
individuals and teachers on
keeping fit. Can refer to local
classes.*

Motability
Goodman House
Station Approach
Harlow
Essex CM20 2ET
Helpline: 0845 456 4566
Tel: 01279 635999
Fax: 01279 632000
Textphone: 01279 632273
Website: www.motability.co.uk
*Advises people with
disabilities about powered
wheelchairs, scooters, and
new and used cars, how to
adapt them to their needs and
obtain funding via the
Mobility Scheme.*

**National Association of
Citizens Advice Bureaux**
see Citizens Advice

New Tax Credit
Department for Work and
Pensions
Palatine House
Lancaster Road
Preston PR1 1HB
Helpline: 0845 300 3900
Tel: 020 7712 2171
Fax: 020 7712 2386
Website: www.dwp.gov.uk
*Government department
giving information about
Working Tax Credit and
Child Tax Credit.*

NHS Direct
Helpline: 0845 4647
Textphone: 0845 606 4647
Tel: 020 8867 1300
Website:
www.nhsdirect.nhs.uk
*A 24-hour helpline offering
confidential health-care
advice, information and
referral service 365 days of
the year. A good first port of
call for any health advice.*

NHS 24 (Scotland)
Tel: 0800 24 24 24
Website: www.nhs24.com
*Scottish 24-hour helpline
offering confidential health-
care advice, information and
referral service 365 days of
the year. A good first port of
call for any health advice.*

NHS Health Scotland
Woodburn House
Canaan Lane
Edinburgh EH10 4SG
Tel: 0131 536 5500
Textphone: 0131 536 5503
Fax: 0131 536 5501
Website:
www.hebs.scot.nhs.uk
*Scotland's NHS health
education board, with some
own leaflets. Has database of
information from other
organisations, to which they
can refer you.*

NHS Smoking Helpline
Helpline: 0800 169 0 169
Website:
www.givingupsmoking.co.uk
*For advice, help and
encouragement on giving up
smoking. Specialist advisers
available to offer on-going
support to those who
genuinely are trying to stop
smoking. Can refer to local
branches.*

**Prescription Pricing
Authority**
PPC Issue Office
PO Box 854
Newcastle upon Tyne NE99
2DE
Advice/Order line: 0845 850
0030
Website: www.ppa.org.uk/ppc
*For information about
prescription charges and the
prepayment certificate.
('season ticket') for
prescriptions.*

**Princess Royal Trust for
Carers**
142 Minories
London EC3N 1LB
Tel: 020 7480 7788
Fax: 020 7481 4729
Website: www.carers.org
*Offers information on a UK-
wide network of independent
carer centres, as well as
advice and support to all
carers. Information available
on website or by telephone.*

GLASGOW OFFICE
Campbell House
215 West Campbell Street
Glasgow G2 4TT
Tel: 0141 221 5066
Fax: 0141 221 4623
Website: www.carers.org

NORTHERN OFFICE
Suite 4, Oak House
High Street
Chorley PR7 1DW
Tel: 01257 234070
Fax: 01257 234105
Website: www.carers.org

Quackwatch
Website: www.quackwatch.org
*A famous American medical
website devoted to debunking
health-related fraud, myths,
fads, fallacies and especially
spurious alternative
treatments and quackery.*

Quit (formerly **Smoking Quitline**)
Ground Floor
211 Old Street
London EC1V 9NR
Helpline: 0800 00 22 00
Tel: 020 7251 1551
Fax: 020 7251 1661
Website: www.quit.org.uk
Offers individual advice on giving up smoking, in English and Asian languages. Talks to schools on smoking and pregnancy, and can refer to local groups. Runs training courses for professionals.

RADAR (Royal Association for Disability and Rehabilitation)
12 City Forum
250 City Road
London EC1V 8AF
Tel: 020 7250 3222
Textphone: 020 7250 4119
Fax: 020 7250 0212
Website: www.radar.org.uk
Campaigns to improve the rights and care of disabled people. Sells special key to access locked public toilets for the disabled.

Royal British Legion
48 Pall Mall
London SW1Y 5JY
Helpline: 0845 772 5725
Tel: 020 7973 7200
Fax: 020 7973 7399
Website:
www.britishlegion.org.uk
Information about possible help for serving and former members of the armed forces and their dependants.

SSAFA Forces Help
(formerly **Soldiers, Sailors and Air Force Association**)
Special Needs Adviser
19 Queen Elizabeth Street
London SE1 2LP
Tel: 020 7403 8783
Fax: 020 7403 8815
Website: www.ssafa.org.uk
National charity offering information, advice and financial aid to serving and ex-service men and women and their families who are in need.

Ulster Cancer Foundation
40–44 Eglantine Avenue
Belfast BT9 6DX
Tel: 028 9066 3281
Fax: 028 9066 0081
Website:
www.ulstercancer.org
Offers advice to help to people wanting to give up smoking.

Index

Note Page numbers in *italics* indicate illustrations and/or instructions for use of devices. Page numbers followed by *g* refer to glossary items.

BRITISH LUNG FOUNDATION

One person in seven in the UK is affected by a lung disease. Whether it's mild asthma or lung cancer, the British Lung Foundation is here for every one of them.

The British Lung Foundation (BLF) relies entirely on voluntary donations, so every gift we receive is a vital contribution towards our fight against lung disease. However, there are other ways you can get involved with BLF; one way is to get involved with our Breathe Easy Groups.

What is Breathe Easy?

Breathe Easy is a support network for people who have a lung condition and for those who look after them. People with lung conditions and those who care for them often feel alone. Making friends is important for people living with lung disease, and Breathe Easy provides a good opportunity for that to happen. The network includes groups that meet in many different towns and cities in the UK. Through events, Breathe Easy works to raise awareness of lung disease and promotes greater understanding of the problems it can cause.

Do I have to pay?

No. If you wish to make a donation you can. Any donation will help people living with lung disease and their carers by providing them with information, support and lung research.

How Breathe Easy can help you

- A quarterly magazine – *Breathing Space*
- Providing free information
- Breathe Easy on-line via the BLF website – www.lunguk.org
- Pen pals scheme

Join a group today!

Breathe Easy is a network of more than 130 groups that run a range of activities, such as regular meetings, social events like trips or tea parties, access to a medical professionals and opportunities to meet, share experiences and find out more about what's going on in the local community.

The British Lung Foundation relies entirely on voluntary donations. Every gift we receive is a vital contribution towards our work. If you can help us, please fill in this form and send it to the address below. Thank you.

Yes, I would like to make a donation of:

☐ £10   ☐ £15   ☐ £30   Other: £ _____ by

☐ Cheque / Postal Order (payable to British Lung Foundation), or

☐ Credit / Debit Card (please circle your choice):

MasterCard / Visa / CAF (Charity Card) / Maestro / Delta

Card no. __ __ __ __ / __ __ __ __ / __ __ __ __ / __ __ __ __ / __ __ __ __

Security no. __ __ __ (last 3 digits on reverse of your card)

Expiry date __ __/__ __   Issue no. _____ (Maestro only)

Cardholder's signature _____ Date ___ / ___ / _____

Please return this form and your gift to:
Appeals Team, British Lung Foundation, FREEPOST SW1233, London EC1B 1BR

Your Details (please use CAPITAL LETTERS):

Title _____   First name _____

Last name _____

Address _____

_____ Postcode _____

Telephone _____ Email _____

We automatically send you an acknowledgement for your gift. If you do not want one, however, please tick here ☐

Gift Aid makes every £1 you give the British Lung Foundation worth £1.28.

☐ Yes, I am a tax payer and I'd like the British Lung Foundation to reclaim the tax on all donations I have made since April 6th 2000 and all future ones, until I notify you otherwise.

☐ No, I am not a UK taxpayer   Date ___ / ___ / _____

Please note: to qualify for Gift Aid, what you pay in income tax or capital gains tax must at least equal the amount we will claim in the tax year.

Before you return your gift, it would be very useful to know why you have decided to support the British Lung Foundation. Please tick one of the following options:

☐ In memory of a relative or friend

☐ In honour of someone's birthday, wedding anniversary, etc.

☐ Other (please give details) _____

Thank you for your feedback, which will help us better understand our supporters.

We may, from time to time, allow certain other charities to contact you. If you would prefer not to receive these communications, please tick here ☐

Have you found **COPD – the 'at your fingertips' guide** useful and practical? If so, you may be interested in other books from Class Publishing.

Asthma – the 'at your fingertips' guide   £17.99
Dr Mark Levy, Trisha Weller and Professor Sean Hilton
Asthma – the 'at your fingertips' guide contains over 250 real questions from people with asthma and their families – answered by three medical experts. This handbook contains up-to-date, medically accurate and practical advice on living with asthma.

> 'A helpful and clearly written book.' – Dr Martyn Partridge, Chief Medical Advisor, National Asthma Campaign

Heart Health – the 'at your fingertips' guide   £14.99
Dr Graham Jackson
This practical handbook, written by a leading cardiologist, answers all your questions about heart conditions. It tells you all about you and your heart; how to keep your heart healthy or – if it has been affected by heart disease – how to make it as strong as possible.

> 'Those readers who want to know more about the various treatments for heart disease will be much enlightened.' – Dr James Le Fanu, The Daily Telegraph

Kidney Failure Explained   £17.99
Dr Andy Stein and Janet Wild
This fully updated new edition of the complete reference manual gives you, your family and friends, the information you really want to know about managing your kidney condition. It also covers recent changes in the health service that will affect the care of people with kidney failure.

> 'This book is, without doubt, the best resource currently available for kidney patients and those who care for them.' – Val Said, kidney transplant patient

Diabetes – the 'at your fingertips' guide   £14.99
Professor Peter Sönksen, Dr Charles Fox and Sue Judd
This is an invaluable reference guide for people with diabetes. It offers practical advice on every aspect of living with the condition, giving you the knowledge and reassurance you need to deal confidently with your diabetes.

> 'I have no hesitation in commending this book.' – Sir Steve Redgrave CBE, Vice President, Diabetes UK

High Blood Pressure – the 'at your fingertips' guide   £14.99
Dr Tom Fahey, Professor Deirdre Murphy with Dr Julian Tudor Hart
The authors use all their years of experience as blood pressure experts to answer your questions on high blood pressure, in order to give you the information you need to bring your blood pressure down – and keep it down.

> 'Readable and comprehensive information' – Dr Sylvia McLaughlan, Director General, The Stroke Association

Beating Depression   £17.99
Dr Stefan Cembrowicz and Dr Dorcas Kingham
Depression is one of most common illnesses in the world – affecting up to one in four people at some time in their lives. *Beating Depression* shows sufferers and their families that they are not alone, and offers tried and tested techniques for overcoming depression.

> 'A sympathetic and understanding guide.' – Marjorie Wallace, Chief Executive, SANE

PRIORITY ORDER FORM

Cut out or photocopy this form and send it (post free in the UK) to:

Class Publishing (London) Ltd
FREEPOST
London W6 7BR

Please send me urgently (*tick below*)	Post included price per copy (*UK only*)
☐ **COPD – the 'at your fingertips' guide** (ISBN 978 1 85959 045 4)	£17.99
☐ **Asthma – the 'at your fingertips' guide** (ISBN 978 1 85959 111 6)	£20.99
☐ **Heart Health – the 'at your fingertips' guide** (ISBN 978 1 85959 097 7)	£17.99
☐ **Kidney Failure Explained** (ISBN 978 1 85959 145 1)	£20.99
☐ **Diabetes – the 'at your fingertips' guide** (ISBN 978 1 85959 087 4)	£17.99
☐ **High Blood Pressure – the 'at your fingertips' guide** (ISBN 978 1 85959 090 4)	£17.99
☐ **Beating Depression** (ISBN 978 1 85959 150 5)	£20.99

TOTAL: _____

Easy ways to pay

Cheque: I enclose a cheque payable to Class Publishing for £_____

Credit card: please debit my ☐ Access ☐ Visa ☐ Amex

Number _____   Expiry date _____

Name _____

My address for delivery is _____

_____

Town _____ County _____ Postcode _____

Telephone number (*in case of query*) _____

Credit card billing address *if different from above* _____

_____

Town _____ County _____ Postcode _____

Class Publishing's guarantee: remember that if, for any reason, you are not satisfied with these books, we will refund all your money, without any questions asked. Prices and VAT rates may be altered for reasons beyond our control.